NEUROTRANSMITTER BALANCES REGULATING BEHAVIOR

NEUROTRANSMITTER BALANCES REGULATING BEHAVIOR

Editors

Edward F. Domino

Department of Pharmacology
University of Michigan
Ann Arbor, Michigan 48104
and
Lafayette Clinic
Detroit, Michigan 48207

and

John M. Davis

Department of Psychiatry
University of Chicago
Chicago, Illinois 60637
and
Illinois State Psychiatric Institute
University of Chicago
Chicago, Illinois 60612

Ann Arbor

International Standard Book Number 0-916182-00-2

Library of Congress Catalog Card Number 75-21131

This book may be purchased from designated bookstores or through P.O. Box 1491, Ann Arbor, Michigan 48106.

Lithographed in U.S.A. by
Edwards Brothers, Inc.
Ann Arbor, Michigan 48104

Officers for 1975
American College of Neuropsychopharmacology, ACNP

Philip R.A. May, M.D.	President
Keith F. Killam, Ph.D.	President-Elect
John J. Burns, Ph.D.	Vice-President
Alberto DiMascio, Ph.D.	Secretary-Treasurer
Seymour Fisher, Ph.D.	Assistant Secretary-Treasurer
Leo E. Hollister, M.D.	Past President

Council

Joseph Cochin, M.D., Ph.D.	Louis Lasagna, M.D.
Leon Epstein, M.D.	Larry Stein, Ph.D.
Donald M. Gallant, M.D.	Leo E. Hollister, M.D.

PREFACE

The origin of this book was a Study Group session of the American College of Neuropsychopharmacology (ACNP) at its annual meeting in San Diego, December 4 to 7, 1973. The ACNP Program Committee for that year approved a session on Neurotransmitters and Autocoid Balances Regulating Behavior. At the time, only abstracts were requested of the participants and these were subsequently published in Psychopharmacology Bulletin, volume 10, number 3, July, 1974 as part of the Abridged Proceedings of the Twelfth Annual Meeting of the ACNP. However, the meeting generated sufficient enthusiasm among the participants that the majority decided to prepare more detailed manuscripts covering their verbal material for this volume. Inasmuch as the ambitious plan to cover both neurotransmitter and autocoid balances was not achieved, the autocoids were dropped and the result is the present title. Two major sessions were held. The first dealt with chemical balances in the brain systems of reward, and the second with neurotransmitter balances in mental illness. Although a few manuscripts were submitted in early 1974, the majority were completed by mid-1975. In a real sense most of the papers record the most recent observations and concepts.

Many of us have become so preoccupied with identifying the behavioral role of a single putative neurotransmitter that we have forgotten the concepts of earlier researchers, such as Hess, who emphasized the antagonistic roles of the ergotropic and tropotropic systems. The trend for looking for complex interactions among neurotransmitters is again becoming more popular. Surely, it will lead to a better understanding of the brain, its chemical mechanisms -- and its function -- behavior.

The efforts of Mrs. Ellen Howard in typing the final manuscripts are gratefully acknowledged.

Edward F. Domino

John M. Davis

October 1, 1975

CONTENTS

CHEMICAL BALANCES IN BRAIN SYSTEMS OF REWARD

NEUROTRANSMITTER BALANCES IN MENTAL DISEASE

CONTENTS

CONTRIBUTORS

George R. Breese, Ph.D.
Departments of Pharmacology
and Psychiatry
University of North Carolina
Chapel Hill, North Carolina 27514

Barrett R. Cooper, Ph.D.
Departments of Pharmacology
and Psychiatry
University of North Carolina
Chapel Hill, North Carolina 27514

John M. Davis, M.D., Ph.D.
Department of Psychiatry
University of Chicago 60637
Chicago, Illinois
and
Illinois State Psychiatric Institute
1601 W. Taylor Street
Chicago, Illinois 60612

Peter B. Dews, Ph.D.
Laboratory of Psychobiology
Harvard Medical School
Boston, Massachusetts 02115

Edward F. Domino, M.D.
Department of Pharmacology
University of Michigan
Ann Arbor, Michigan 48104
and
Laboratory of Pharmacology
The Lafayette Clinic
951 E. Lafayette
Detroit, Michigan 48207

William E. Fann, M.D.
Department of Psychiatry
Baylor University Medical Center
Houston, Texas 77025

Samuel Gershon, M.D.
Department of Psychiatry
New York University Medical School
550 First Avenue
New York, New York 10016

Murray Glusman, M.D.
Columbia University
New York, New York 10032
and
Department of Mental Hygiene
New York State Psychiatric Institute
New York, New York 10032

David S. Janowsky, M.D.
Department of Psychiatry
University of California at San Diego
La Jolla, California 92037

Dennis D. Kelly, Ph.D.
Department of Psychiatry
Columbia University
New York, New York 10032
and
New York State Psychiatric Institute
New York, New York 10032

C. Raymond Lake, M.D., Ph.D.
Department of Psychiatry
Duke University Medical School
P.O. Box 3812
Durham, North Carolina 27710

Lewis R. Mandel, Ph.D.
Department of Biochemistry
Merck Institute for Therapeutic Research
Rahway, New Jersey 07065

Steven Matthysse, Ph.D.
Department of Psychiatry
Harvard Medical School
Boston, Massachusetts 02124

Gerald M. McKenzie, Ph.D.
Wellcome Research Laboratories
3030 Cornwallis Road
Research Triangle Park, North Carolina 27709

Francis W. Ninteman, B.S.
Department of Pharmacology
Research Division
Parke Davis and Company
Ann Arbor, Michigan 48106

B. Paul H. Poschel, Ph.D.
Department of Pharmacology
Research Division
Parke Davis and Company
Ann Arbor, Michigan 48106

S.N. Pradhan, M.D.
Department of Pharmacology
Howard University
College of Medicine
Washington, D.C. 20001

Baron Shopsin, M.D.
Department of Psychiatry
Neuropsychopharmacology Research Unit
New York University School of Medicine
New York, New York 10016

Larry Stein, Ph.D.
Department of Psychopharmacology
Wyeth Laboratories
Philadelphia, Pennsylvania 19101

C. David Wise, Ph.D.
Department of Psychopharmacology
Wyeth Laboratories
Philadelphia, Pennsylvania 19101

Neurotransmitter Balances Regulating Behavior, edited and published by E.F. Domino and J.M. Davis, Ann Arbor, © 1975

PSYCHOANALYTIC CONCEPTS AND BRAIN STIMULATION: A CONSIDERATION OF RELEVANCE

Murray Glusman
Columbia University
and
New York State Psychiatric Institute
New York, New York

Based on their studies of brain stimulation in animals, Stein and Wise (1971) and Wise and Stein (1973) have proposed an interesting biochemical theory concerning the etiology of schizophrenia. They point to the accumulation of research in the past two decades that suggests the existence of two neural systems in the brain, one associated with reward and the other with punishment. The notion of the "reward system" is based on the demonstration that electrical stimulation of certain regions of the brain can serve as a positive reinforcement, a phenomenon first discovered by Olds and Milner (1954). The "punishment system" is based on the demonstration by Delgado *et al*. (1954) that electrical stimulation of certain brain regions in animals is aversive. The reward system, according to the authors, is mainly noradrenergic (Stein, 1971) whereas the punishment system is cholinergic and perhaps serotonergic as well.

Stein and Wise (1971) have proposed that the cause of schizophrenia in man is due to damage to the noradrenergic reward system by the formation of endogenous 6-hydroxydopamine (6-OHDA) as the result of a genetically determined enzymatic error. They note that systematic family studies and studies of adopted children have established the importance of genetic factors in the development of schizophrenia beyond any real doubt (Heston, 1970). The hereditary transmission of schizophrenia involves transmission of a biochemical abnormality, the result of a pathological gene; this results in an enzymatic derangement which permits the formation of 6-OHDA. It was proposed that by some error of enzymatic regulation of norepinephrine metabolism, excessive amounts of dopamine may accumulate in the noradrenergic vesicles and be transformed to 6-OHDA by an autooxidative process or an enzymatic reaction. They suggested the possibility that dopamine-β-hydroxylase might be involved in the enzymatic error (Stein *et al*., 1972). It was also speculated that small amounts of dopamine *o*-quinone

(DOQ) may be formed from dopamine by dopamine-β-hydroxylase and 6-OHDA is formed from the DOQ.

Basic to the Stein and Wise hypothesis is Sandor Rado's psychoanalytic concept which attributes the fundamental defect in schizophrenia to an innate deficiency in the organizing action of pleasure or an "integrative pleasure deficiency" (Rado, 1953; Rado et al., 1956).

Because of the importance attached to Rado's formulations, it would seem useful to review his concepts concerning pleasure and pain, examining their origins and reviewing his formulations on schizophrenia and psychopathology.

Sandor Rado was born in Hungary in 1890. He entered the University of Budapest in 1907, planning at first to study political science and law but after reading a paper by Ferenczi entitled "Analysis of the Soul" he became intensely interested in psychoanalysis and decided that after completing his doctorate in political science he would study medicine, then psychiatry, and devote himself completely to psychoanalysis. After completing his medical studies, he undertook training in psychoanalysis and was analyzed by Karl Abraham, then Director of the Berlin Psychoanalytic Institute (Jameson and Klein, 1969). Rado soon became active in psychoanalytic circles. He became a close friend of Ferenczi and in 1924 at Freud's invitation he became the executive director of the two official psychoanalytic journals: Internationale Zeitschrit für Psychoanalyse and Imago, Zeitschrift für Anwendung der Psychoanalyse auf die Natur und Geisteswissenschaften (Rado, 1948). In 1930 he came to the United States at the invitation of the New York Psychoanalytic Society to help set up the New York Psychoanalytic Institute on the model of the Berlin Psychoanalytic Institute. Rado had a close working relationship with Freud but a rift developed which at first may have been personal but by 1939 Rado was voicing some sharp theoretical differences with Freud's theory of instincts or libido theory. He announced that the factual findings of psychoanalysis must be separated from what he regarded as a kind of Freudian mysticism. In keeping with his view that psychoanalysis should be part of medicine he claimed that it was necessary to build a conceptual frame of reference based on biology.

Rado's comments generated considerable opposition in psychoanalytic circles and 1941 he resigned his position as Director of the New York Psychoanalytic Institute. Soon thereafter, he made a great step toward achieving one of his fondest and most cherished ambitions which was to identify psychoanalysis with medicine. In 1944 he organized the Columbia University Psychoanalytic Clinic for Training and Research within the structure of the Columbia University College of Physicians and Surgeons and as part of the Department of Psychiatry.

Since the psychoanalytic movement in Europe had evolved outside university settings, Rado's achievement in having a psychoanalytic training center established under the auspices of Columbia University was an unusual accomplishment and he was extremely proud of it, feeling that the university affiliation was a sign of medical, scientific and intellectual acceptance. A course of instruction was organized and in addition to Rado's own lectures on adaptational psychodynamics, the term he adopted for his views on psychoanalytic theory, lectures were given on Freud's writings and, at Rado's insistence, some rather unusual courses were included in the curriculum; neurophysiology, taught by Harry Grundfest; neurochemistry, by Heinrich Waelsch; clinical psychiatry, by Paul Hoch; genetics in psychiatry, by Franz Kallmann; and neuropathology, by Armando Ferraro (Rado, 1948).

These courses reflected his own deep interest and respect for the biological sciences. Nevertheless, he had no real working acquaintance with any of the scientific disciplines.

I was privileged to be one of Rado's last students at Columbia before his retirement - and to be taught by him was a most interesting and memorable experience. Rado was a man of short physical stature, but this was more than counterbalanced by his intellectual stature. He had a vast amount of energy, a tremendous enthusiasm for his topic; he was intellectually very gifted, and he enjoyed enormously dealing with concepts, theories, and abstractions on a grand scale. He was a witty man and at times caustic, and he applied a blend of the two with enormous zest and devastating effect to one of his favorite tasks, which was demolishing Freudian libido theory. He felt that the important role that Freud assigned to instincts as motivating forces in behavior was utter nonsense and that libido theory had evolved into an obscure blend of animism and mysticism - totally removed from science and logic.

To underscore his point, he would recount to his students, with relish and delight, Hans Christian Andersen's story of the Emperor's New Clothes (Andersen, 1945). The Emperor, who was excessively fond of fine clothing, was convinced by a pair of fraudulent weavers that they could create for him the most unimaginably fine and magnificent clothes. Not only was the fabric beautiful beyond belief - it had the extraordinary property of being invisible to anyone who was impossibly stupid or otherwise unworthy of his office.

Taken in by the story, the Emperor, for a handsome sum, engaged the weavers to make him these remarkable new clothes. The weavers set to work pretending to weave the fabric which was invisible because it was non-existent. The Emperor and his courtiers praised the remarkable beauty of the "cloth," distrusting the evidence of their eyes and senses, and not daring to confess they could see nothing at all. Such an admission, after all, would be tantamount to a confession of stupidity or incompetence or both. Eventually, when the remarkable clothes were finished, the Emperor, clad only in the non-existent, imaginary garments displayed them in a grand parade before his assembled subjects. The spectators gasped and marveled at their beauty, none daring to admit they could see no clothes until a little child cried that the Emperor had nothing on. From person to person the child's words swept until at last the great hoax was exposed and all the spectators roared that the Emperor was without clothes.

Rado no doubt saw himself as the heroic child who, by trusting his mind and senses, exposed a great hoax, revealing libido theory to be devoid of substance and nothing more than an elaborate figment of the imagination.

Having rejected Freudian instincts as the prime motivating forces of behavior, he was faced with the necessity of finding some logical and scientifically rational alternative. What he did was to formulate his conceptual scheme "Adaptational Psychodynamics" (Rado, 1956). To do this he turned to some great scientific contributions and to some important philosophical ideas.

Rado was fascinated by science, but not on the level of the grubby details of the laboratory bench; his interest was in the great scientific theories and generalizations - he was attracted by the clear logic, the rationality, and the authority of science. Thus, although he knew little about neurology, he was a great admirer of Hughlings Jackson's notions of hierarchical levels in the nervous system (Jackson, 1958); he knew little about physiology, but he was fascinated with Walter Cannon's interest in fear and rage (Cannon, 1953), and Cannon's ideas on homeostasis (Cannon, 1939); he knew little of biology, but he was intimately concerned with Darwin and evolution (Darwin, 1950, 1955). His fascination with science was not an idle one; he incorporated Jackson's ideas as well as Darwin's and Cannon's into his own formulations.

Rado was also greatly interested in philosophy; he had his Ph.D. in Political Science and he was quite familiar with a group of philosophers who were as important for their ideas on politics as for their contributions to philosophy. Among them were Jeremy Bentham (1748-1832) and his school who derived their major philosophical orientation - which came to be called "Utilitarianism" - from Locke, Hartley and Helvétius. Bentham and his followers, who included James Mill and his son, John Stuart Mill, became the leaders of British radicalism. Eventually their school - the Philosophical Radicals - gave rise to Socialism and Darwinism.

Bentham, who was interested in ethics and politics (Bentham, 1939), based his philosophy on two principles: the association principle and the greatest happiness principle. The association principle was derived from a predecessor, Hartley, but Bentham made it a basic principle of psychology, recognizing the association of ideas and language, as well as the association of ideas and ideas (Russell, 1945).

Bentham's goal was to establish a legal code and a social system that would make men virtuous. To define virtue he had to introduce his greatest happiness principle, maintaining that what is good is pleasure or happiness and what is bad is pain. "Therefore, one state of affairs is better than another if it involves a greater balance of pleasure over pain, or a smaller balance of pain over pleasure. The best possible state of affairs is the one involving the greatest balance of pleasure over pain (Russell, 1945, p. 775)."

Bentham and his followers applied their doctrines to practical politics and the Benthamites had a great influence on British legislation and policy in the middle of the nineteenth century.

Like Bentham and the utilitarians, Rado placed major emphasis on pleasure and pain. Bentham, however, was con-concerned with guiding principles in the political sphere; Rado made pleasure and pain the cornerstones of organismic behavior. He proposed what he called a "central integrative apparatus" (in the psychocerebral system or mind) and, in line with Hughlings Jackson's notion of hierarchical levels of organization in the brain (Jackson, 1958), derived as a result of evolution, Rado proposed a somewhat similar arrangement for the "central integrative apparatus" with four major subdivisions or levels arranged around a common axis (Rado, 1964). The oldest and most primitive level, the level of hedonic self-regulation, is seen phylogenetically in protozoa and it entails the self-regulatory system which makes the organism move toward a source of pleasure and away from a source of pain. He felt that the organism's systemic requirements generate various tensions, urges and needs which prompt the organism to action to supply the various needs. The organism then in its contact with the environment is guided by responses of pleasure and pain. Pleasure becomes a reward for successful performance and memory of pleasure prompts repetition of the successful activity. Conversely, pain becomes punishment for failure and memory of pain deters the organism from repeating injurious activity. The next higher level in the remaining hierarchical levels of the psychodynamic cerebral system is the "preverbal level of brute emotion" which is dominated by two classes of emotions: The welfare emotions - such as pleasurable desire, joy, affection, love and pride; these are all variants of pleasure. Then there are the emergency emotions - agony, fear, rage, retroflexed rage, guilty fear, and guilty rage - all related to the experience or expectation of pain. The emergency emotions, in line with Cannon's ideas, prepare the organism for flight or combat and take precedence over all other motivations.

The next higher level is emotional thought and finally the highest level is unemotional thought. The emotional thought level culminates in religion, art, and aesthetic pleasure; unemotional thought in science, technology and wisdom.

Hedonic self-regulation involves all the phases of organization from the lowest to the highest. So that just as the infant operates on the basis of primitive pleasure and pain, so the highest levels of an adult's intellectual activities entail expectations of delayed reward instead of immediate reward - or expected disapproval instead of immediate pain as on the lower levels.

The organism's awareness of itself develops via proprioceptive sensations. Thus, an infant in becoming aware of his own muscular activity develops an awareness of himself as the one who acts. Self-awareness develops from the "action-self" which is the organism's highest decision-making unit. The "action-self" occupies a central position in each of the hierarchical levels (Rado, 1964).

Rado accepted Kallmann's suggestion of a genetic basis for schizophrenia (Kallmann, 1938). The schizophrenic genotype, that is, an individual with a genetic predisposition to schizophrenia, he felt manifested a particular kind of psychodynamic picture which he called the schizotypal organization. Thus, Rado (1953) said: "In the schizotypes the machinery of psychodynamic integration is strikingly inadequate, because one of its essential components, the organizing action of pleasure - its motivational strength - is innately defective [p. 411]." His phrase for this crucial defect was "integrative pleasure deficiency." Sometimes, patients recognize this and will say about themselves that they are incapable of giving and sharing love.

The basic difficulty in the inadequacy of the welfare emotions creates major problems. The welfare emotions counterbalance the emergency emotions and since in schizotypes the welfare emotions are weak or inadequate, this causes an emotional imbalance so that the emergency emotions tend to grow excessive and schizotypes show unusually intense fear and unusually intense rage. The deficiency in the integrative aspects of pleasure impairs the individual's development of the "action-self." Thus, Rado (1953) commented: "pleasure is the tie that really binds [p. 411]," and, therefore, an action-self without the strong integrative aspect of pleasure is weak and prone to break under stress. The weakness of the action-self is evidenced by the patient's oversensitivity and profound insecurity about himself, his body and his environment. The impaired capacity for pleasure and love prevents healthy sexual function. The sexual organization lacks genuine love and tenderness and is prone to fragmentation. The individual evolves a scarcity economy of pleasure and a security pattern marked by compensatory dependence. Sometimes behavior which is ordinarily handled simply and automatically on the basis of pleasurable feeling is carried out by unemotional thought (Rado, 1953). In similar fashion, Rado derived many aspects of schizophrenic behavior from the basic weakness in pleasure or the welfare emotions.

Rado's views on adaptional psychodynamics and schizophrenia are important and worth serious examination. He extended the views on pleasure and pain of the Utilitarian School of philosophers from the social and political sphere to the psychological sphere. Then, utilizing the scientific contributions of Hughlings Jackson, Darwin and Walter Cannon, he synthesized a psychological system to explain human behavior, both normal and disordered. It is interesting that despite his great concern with scientific contributions in many fields, he tended to overlook the contributions of modern psychology. He made no mention of C. Lloyd Morgan or Thorndike and took little or no notice of Watson, Pavlov, Skinner, Hull, Spence, Hebb, Neal Miller or the ethologists. His concern was with subjective, introspectional phenomena in man and he had little interest in the powerful trends in psychology that dismissed subjective phenomena and focused on behaviorism. There could be little attraction for Rado in the credo expressed by Watson (1913):

> Psychology as the behaviorist views it is a purely objective experimental branch of natural science. Its theoretical goal is the prediction

> and control of behavior. Introspection forms no essential part of its methods, nor is the scientific value of its data dependent upon the readiness with which they lend themselves to interpretation in terms of consciousness... [p. 158]. The time seems to have come when psychology must discard all reference to consciousness; when it need no longer delude itself into thinking that is is making mental states the object of observation...[p. 163]. Psychology, as the behaviorist views it, is a purely objective, experimental branch of natural science which needs introspection as little as do the sciences of chemistry and physics [p. 176].

Also, despite his great interest in science and the philosophy of science - he referred repeatedly to Mach, Poincaré, Nernst, Reichenbach, v.Mises, Bridgman and Woodger - he made little use of scientific method. He was not concerned with systematic observation, acquisition of data, experimental manipulation and hypothesis testing - in short with the indispensable procedures and tools of the empirical scientist. Thus, the principles he derived and the theories he propounded, reasonable and rational as they were, were basically speculations which lacked an empirical base in the subject they dealt with. It is interesting too, that for all of Rado's criticism of Freud and for all of Rado's interest in science, Freud made significant efforts to build his ideas on an empirical foundation, utilizing data from case histories, dream material, and free associations; whereas Rado made no such effort. Rado's relationship to science was in a sense, second hand; he worked with the principles and generalizations that others had derived in various fields and used them as the basis for a set of theoretical constructs dealing with psychopathology. Rado's tools were the philosopher's tools, the power of his own intellect and an admirable ability to reason logically and clearly. With those tools he built an important set of theories concerning human behavior and psychopathology.

The question to be asked now is how relevant are these concepts to brain stimulation? Stein and Wise have felt that they are extremely relevant, even constructing a theory concerning the biochemical disturbance in schizophrenia which relates directly to Rado's concepts. It should be pointed out that Rado's ideas cannot enhance the validity of Stein and Wise's hypothesis because Rado's notions, as indicated in detail above, are in the final analysis, speculations rooted in philosophical notions and thus far they are unsupported by scientific data or evidence. Stein and Wise's theory provides an interesting extension and elaboration of Rado's theory, but a theory based upon a theory is a tenuous creation at best. Still, no matter how insubstantial the grounds on which a theory rests, there is no logical reason why it may not prove to be correct, and if not correct it may nevertheless stimulate important research and lead to valuable discoveries. Stein and Wise have pointed out that the neural pathways involved in self-stimulation appear to be chiefly noradrenergic whereas the "punishment" system appears to be at least partly serotonergic. They suggest that the pathways involved in self-stimulation constitute the chief reward or pleasure system of the brain and that damage to the noradrenergic terminals of this system via the endogenous formation of 6-OHDA produced by DOQ results in impairment of the pleasure system of the brain, loss of its integrative action, and production of schizophrenia in accordance with Rado's hypothesis. Most recently, Wise and Stein (1973, 1975) have reported that, in line with their hypothesis, dopamine-β-hydroxylase activity is significantly reduced in the brains of schizophrenic patients compared to normals.

Ultimately, the validity of this hypothesis must be established on biochemical grounds; nevertheless, from the standpoint of Rado's concepts, some questions must be clarified.

The obvious and inescapable problem which arises in attempting to relate Stein and Wise's brain stimulation studies with Rado's psychoanalytic concepts is the problem of anthropomorphization. Rado quite clearly pointed out that we know about subjective feeling states via communicated introspection (Rado, 1962):

> Although introspection is a private operation of one individual, he can communicate the products of this operation to a participant observer. If, for instance, a patient tells me that he is 'happy' or 'angry' or 'afraid,' I understand what he means because I have experienced these feelings myself and have learned to associate the feelings with words. In order to understand communicated introspection, each of us must use his own introspection as a model, a mediating referent [p. 154].

Communicated introspection is obviously out of the question in animal studies. To obviate the problem of anthropomorphization, the "reward system" and the "punishment system" were defined operationally. Unlike other systems which have clearly defined functional, neuroanatomical and neurophysiological relationships such as the visual system, the auditory system, the somatosensory system and the motor system, the "reward" and "punishment" systems owe their existence to operational definitions. Operational definitions may be very useful for experimental purposes; they may be of great help in studying various aspects of self-stimulation, or the aversive properties of intracranial stimulation; they guard against the temptation for egregious anthropomorphization; but they leave unanswered the functional significance of the operationally defined systems. Further, too, the relationship of the operationally defined system to known, conventional systems may be confusing and overlapping. For example, if an animal finds stimulation of a given site aversive and works to avoid or escape the stimulus, we are evidently justified in including the locus in the "punishment system." But an animal will find electrical stimulation of the cornea or tooth-pulp aversive. By our operational definition the cornea and tooth-pulp would be included in the "punishment system," although the cornea is, of course, part of the visual system and teeth are primarily involved in feeding and attack or defense. Pain can be elicited from almost any bodily region and there is a considerable body of information concerning the psychological neuroanatomical and neurophysiological aspects of pain; but the relationship between the conventional pain system and the "punishment system" is unclear and confusing. Does the punishment system exist as a separate entity? Does it overlap the pain system, or is it merely an operationally defined portion of centrally coursing pain pathways?

The "reward system" poses similar problems. The discovery of the phenomenon of self-stimulation by Olds and Milner in 1954 initiated a flood of investigations. The phenomenon has been replicated in numerous species and a great deal of information has been gathered concerning the rewarding properties of brain stimulation. Still, the fundamental significance of the "reward system" is far from clear. Almost all of the information available concerning the "reward system" comes from animal studies and again we are confronted with the problem of anthropomorphization. Some limited information has been gleaned from depth-electrode studies in humans by a handful of investigators, but that information is incomplete and inconclusive. Ethical, moral and legal sanctions against human experimentation make it difficult, if not impossible, to determine the significance of the "reward system" in man.

The questions that must be answered concerning the

"reward system" are: First, what significance does the system have for the subjective emotional experience of pleasure in man? Then, to what extent is the "system" a system in the conventional sense, in that it constitutes an anatomically and physiologically related entity whose function is to subserve all pleasure, whether it be from ingestion of food, sex, pleasure of achievement, etc.? Also, is the system so interrelated and unified structurally that it can be destroyed by anatomical or chemical means, and, if destroyed, will a person so afflicted manifest partial or even complete inability to experience pleasure from any and all sources?

The information available to date in man - well reviewed by Valenstein (1973) - is too fragmentary to answer these questions. What we know comes largely from the observations by Heath and his associates at Tulane (Heath and Mickle, 1960; Bishop _et al._, 1963; Heath, 1963, 1964, 1972; Heath _et al._, 1968), Sem-Jacobsen and Torkildsen (1960), Sem-Jacobsen (1968), and Bechterewa (1969). Brain stimulation at some sites in humans evidently can produce feelings of well-being or pleasure. One of Heath's patients had attempted suicide, but shortly after the attempt when an electrode in his septal region was stimulated he announced that he felt good although it was difficult for him to explain why he felt good (Valenstein, 1973). A woman with intractable pain said that the stimulus made her feel fine and energetic. In some instances patients may have experienced sexual orgasms during brain stimulation. These may or may not have been secondary to sensations in the genitalia produced by the stimulus. Humans may self-stimulate but for unexpected reasons. One of Heath's patients kept trying to recall a memory vaguely elicited by the stimulus. Heath (1963) reported:

> The button most frequently pushed provided a stimulus to the centromedian thalamus. This stimulus did not, however, induce the most pleasurable response; in fact, it induced irritability. The subject reported that he was almost able to recall a memory during this stimulation, but he could not quite grasp it. The frequent self-stimulations were an endeavor to bring this elusive memory into clear focus [p. 573, 574].

Sem-Jacobsen (1968) described similar reasons for self-stimulation with the patients trying to clarify the nature of a fleeting or puzzling sensation. He commented:

> An emotional reward often has been designated as an explanation or motivation for self-

> stimulation; an unpleasant response is thought to cause the patient to avoid stimulation. In humans, however, other incentives are also very strong and can sometimes be more potent than the simple pleasure received. The reasons given by patients for continuing self-stimulation seem as complex as man himself. In man, curiosity is probably the most dominant causative factor in initiating self-stimulation [p. 54].

He noted too, that a pleasurable response is at times secondary to muscular contractions in the region of the genitals. Thus, Sem-Jacobsen and Torkildsen (1960) observed:

> In secluded patients it is difficult to evaluate whether the change in mood is a result of central stimulation or a central effect of peripheral reactions to the stimulus. For instance, one patient laughed with joy in response to each stimulation. After several days with stimulation we learned what really took place. The stimulus evoked a fluttering in a muscle group in the pelvis which tickled the patient and she responded with joy and laughter [p. 284].

Bechterewa (1969) reported several instances in which brain stimulation in patients produced pleasurable, erotic sensations and in one woman they led to orgasm (p. 165). Self-stimulation has been reported in humans but great care is required in interpreting the response. Thus, Bishop _et al_. (1963) and Brazier (1964) noted instances in which patients continued to "self-stimulate" for long periods even after the current had been turned off. Bishop _et al_'s patient was a catatonic schizophrenic with marked perseverative behavior. His perseverative tendency included lever-pressing in the self-stimulation study, complicating the study greatly because he lever-pressed with current on or off.

Clearly, much more needs to be known about both the "reward system" and "punishment system" in man before we can understand their significance. But even if we were to assume with Stein and Wise that there did indeed exist a unified reward or pleasure system in the brain, what evidence would we have that impairment of the system is a central factor in schizophrenia? Rado emphasized anhedonia in schizophrenia and made it a basic feature of that disorder. But Rado did not base his conclusions on systemically collected empirical data; his collected papers include only one clinical investigation (Rado _et al_., 1956) which consisted of a preliminary report of an elaborate, diffuse, clinical study that was never completed and which in no way proved his contention that anhedonia is a crucial element in schizophrenia. Rado himself cited Bleuler as authority for the importance of anhedonia in schizophrenia:

> Beginning with Bleuler, clinical observers have repeatedly listed 'anhedonia' and 'proprioceptive disorder' among the symptoms of schizophrenia. In contradistinction, the aforesaid inherited defects are viewed here not merely as symptoms, but as the _two central axes of an organization sui generis_ (Rado _et al._, 1956, p. 226).

But Bleuler made no mention of anhedonia; he stressed disturbance of affect. The schizophrenic may, of course, be anhedonic; flattening of affect is a common enough feature in schizophrenia, but flattening of affect encompasses much more and is a broader and more inclusive disturbance than anhedonia. It is, of course, by no means uncommon to find schizophrenics who are quite capable of experiencing pleasure, although the pleasure may be strikingly inappropriate to the circumstances which elicit it.

Thus, for example, Bleuler (1950) stated:

> Especially conspicuous in schizophrenics is the frequently encountered parathymia. The patients are able to react to sad news with cheerfulness or even with laughter. These patients will often become sad, or even more frequently, irritated by events to which others would react with indifference or with pleasure...In the fields of taste and smell, the parathymic disturbance can often be very prominent...A catatonic whom I asked why he drank his own urine, answered with a blissfully entranced expression, 'Herr Direktor, if you should taste it but once, you would never want to drink anything else' [p. 52].

Clearly the patient cited by Bleuler was capable of experiencing pleasure; he was not at all anhedonic but his pleasure, to say the least, was grossly unusual and highly inappropriate.

Actually, anhedonia is not a very common term; it is not listed in the Oxford English Dictionary (1961) or the American Heritage Dictionary (1973), nor can it be found in the indexes of such widely used texts of psychiatry as Kolb's (Noyes' Modern Clinical Psychiatry, 1968), Freedman and Kaplan's (Comprehensive Textbook of Psychiatry, 1967), or Arieti's (American Handbook of Psychiatry, 1974). But it is listed in Webster's Third New International Dictionary (1968) where it is defined as "1. Insensitiveness to pleasure. 2. Incapacity for experiencing happiness." It is a curious thing that the term never achieved wide popularity in psychiatry and when it is mentioned, as in Meehl (1962) it tends to be related to Rado and his theory concerning schizophrenia. It is odd, too, that the term anhedonia is generally not applied to depressive states although it would seem to be eminently applicable to depressed patients. To be depressed and to be able to experience pleasure is virtually a contradiction in terms. Only when the depressed patient begins to recover does he regain his capacity to experience happiness, but while he is depressed and for the duration of his depression he is by definition anhedonic, and the term is as applicable to him as to any schizophrenic.

To consider another point, Rado pointed out that pleasure and the welfare emotions counterbalance the pain-connected emergency emotions; hence:

> In the schizotypes, motivational weakness of the welfare emotions causes an emotional disbalance; without this adequate tempering influence the emergency emotions tend to grow excessive in motivational strength and integrative scope [Rado, 1953, p. 411].

Thus, the schizotypes show greatly exaggerated fear and rage responses.

As for fear and rage responses, Reis, Gunne and their associates (Reis et al., 1967; Gunne, 1969) have obtained evidence in cats indicating that the central mechanisms mediating rage responses produced either by brain stimulation or high decerebration involve noradrenergic pathways. Hence, impairment of noradrenergic nerve terminals should interfere with fear and rage, reducing the emergency emotions as well as pleasure and the welfare emotions. If the motivational weakness due to impairment of the emergency emotions is added to the motivational weakness of the welfare emotions the expected clinical picture resulting from impairment of noradrenergic pathways should show a striking loss of motivation. Since there is also evidence that feeding behavior is noradrenergically mediated (Leibowitz, 1974) there should be loss of appetite as well. Loss of interest in sex should be included too since Stein (1971) suggested that sexual activity is included in the reward system. He commented:

> Briefly, electrical stimulation of the medial forebrain bundle serves as a powerful reward and also elicits species-typical consummatory

> responses, such as feeding and copulation, which produce pleasure and permit satisfaction of basic needs [p. 346].

From the above, the clinical picture to be expected from damage to the noradrenergic nerve terminals should include among its key features loss of pleasurable responses or impaired gratification, reduced fear and rage, impaired motivation, impaired appetite and loss of interest in sex. This constellation of symptoms corresponds much more closely with the most prominent features of depressive states than with those of schizophrenia.

Beck (1967) in a study of 966 psychiatric patients found some degree of sadness or unhappiness in 88 per cent of severely depressed patients compared with 23 per cent of non-depressed patients.

Loss of gratification was the most prominent complaint. He reported:

> The loss of gratification is such a pervasive process among depressives that many patients regard it as the central feature of their illness. In our series, 92 per cent of the severely depressed patients reported at least partial loss of satisfaction; this was the most common symptom among the depressed group as a whole [p. 18].

Loss of positive motivation was found in 86 per cent of Beck's severely depressed patients and in 65 per cent of the mildly depressed ones.

> The loss of positive motivation is often a striking feature of depression. The patient may have a major problem in mobilizing himself to perform even the most elemental and vital tasks as eating, elimination, or taking medication to relieve his distress [p. 27].

Anorexia is also one of the most common features of depression. It was found in 72 per cent of severely depressed patients compared to 21 per cent of nondepressed patients. "For many patients loss of appetite is often the first sign of an incipient depression and return of appetite may be the first sign that it is beginning to lift [Beck, 1967, p. 33]." Lastly, there was some loss of interest in sex either autoerotic or heterosexual in 61 per cent of the depressed patients and only 27 per cent of nondepressed patients. In severely depressed patients "Any responsiveness to sexual stimuli is lost and the patients may have a pronounced aversion for sex [Beck, 1967, p. 35]."

Aggression bears a somewhat special relationship to depression. On a hospital ward the severely depressed patient is not an assaultive, violent, combative individual; he can barely mobilize himself to carry on the everyday tasks of getting dressed, washing, eating, etc. Thus, during severe depressive states aggressive behavior is decreased and the depressed patient is a most unaggressive individual. However, as the patient begins to recover from his depression, aggressive behavior may appear as violence directed against the self in suicide, or as suicide combined with homicide, in which the patient may destroy himself and one or more members of his immediate family; _e.g._, a husband may not only kill himself, but his wife and children as well, whom he may regard as extensions of himself.

All in all, a strong case can be made that there is a better fit between Stein and Wise's hypothesis with depression than with schizophrenia. There is, of course, a considerable body of evidence implicating noradrenergic mechanisms in depressive states; much of this information has been summarized by Schildkraut (1965), Schildkraut _et al_. (1965), and Schildkraut and Kety (1967) as part of the catecholamine hypothesis of affective disorders. Stein and Wise's notions may be regarded as a further theoretical contribution to the catecholamines hypothesis. A particularly valuable addition to the hypothesis may be their suggestion (Stein _et al_., 1972) that after damage to the noradrenergic nerve terminals denervation supersensitivity to norepinephrine may develop. The development of denervation supersensitivity provides a most interesting possibility for explaining the cyclical nature of some affective disorders, _e.g._, manic-depressive states.

Clearly, we still have not achieved a reasonable hypothesis for the neurochemical basis of schizophrenia. The dopamine hypothesis for the etiology of schizophrenia elaborated by Snyder (1974) and Matthysse (1973), based on findings by Carlsson and Lindqvist (1963) has generated a good deal of interest among investigators in psychiatry. By and large, it seems more defensible than Stein and Wise's hypothesis. Nevertheless, its validity is far from established.

The catecholamine hypothesis for the affective disorders, the Stein and Wise hypothesis and the dopamine hypothesis for schizophrenia may all have their shortcomings; it is heartening, nevertheless, to note that with the rapid expansion of research in the neurosciences we are acquiring sufficiently detailed information concerning brain function to develop increasingly sophisticated and meaningful theories concerning the etiology of some major psychiatric disorders. Not very long ago the possibility of relating the etiology of schizophrenia and the affective disorders to the brain seemed unattainably remote. Currently, as research in psychopharmacology moves with increasing direction and sophistication to the level of the neurotransmitters, there are occasional clues that we may be moving in the right direction and that we may find the answers to the etiology of schizophrenia and the affective disorders in the not too distant future.

To conclude, Rado would have been immensely pleased to know that his formulations were sufficiently relevant to provide physiologists and biochemists with important clues for research in schizophrenia. Since he was an excellent logician he would have recognized that building a theory on a theory is a precarious venture at best. Nevertheless, as he maintained again and again to his students - theories are not dogma; they are made to be broken; what is important about a theory is that it makes new advances possible and that it stimulates new research. And that, of course, is what Rado's own concepts and Stein and Wise's ideas seem to be doing.

Little has been said about Freud in this presentation because of the problem of relating Freudian psychoanalytic theory to brain physiology. Rado (1962) saw the difficulty clearly and elucidated it in the following manner:

> Freud, the pioneer, took no time out for methodological considerations. He did not realize, nor did anyone else for quite some time, that during the development of his basic theory of the structure and function of the mind he gradually switched from a mechanistic to an animistic conceptual scheme. The shift began in 1905, with the introduction of his Theory of Instincts (the Libido theory, subsequently elaborated into the Theory of Eros and the death instincts), and climaxed, in the 1920s, in the transformation of the concept of 'mental apparatus' into the tripartite structural notion of superego, ego and id. Brain physiology, like all physiology, is mechanistic. While Freud's originally mechanistic theory offered hope for correlation with brain physiology, his later animistic notions did not. Consequently, psychoanalysis became separated from human biology. In the last two decades, more and more people have felt that psychoanalysis was 'on the loose.' Instead of examining the question why, some writers suggested that psychoanalytic

> theory be viewed and cultivated as a social science.
>
> Ancient man was animistic. Analyzing his sensory experience in the relation of cause and effect, he attributed natural events to the action of man-like creatures hiding behind them. In the early nineteenth century vitalistic biology--thinly disguised animism--traced human behavior to the action of vital spirits hiding in the ventricles of the brain. Instinct, superego, ego and id are these old vital spirits reintroduced into psychoanalytic theory; the core of each is a miniature personage. To explain *homo* by making him appear as an organization of *homunculi* is a classical instance of the well-known logical fallacy of *petitio principii*; no wonder, animistic (vitalistic) theories have proved unworkable. The life sciences have become what they now are by advancing from the animistic to the mechanistic model [p. 179-180].

To some extent Freud's problem may have been the fact that he began his career as a neurologist. Knowing more about the brain than Rado and seeing it through the eyes of a nineteenth century neurologist, he viewed the task of relating psychiatric disturbances to the chemistry and physiology of the brain as being so far removed as to be almost hopelessly in the future. Thus, he went on to develop psychoanalysis, libido theory and a frame of reference which is very difficult to relate to modern neurophysiology and neurochemistry.

Freud, nevertheless, always felt that the answers to mental illness would eventually come from the laboratories of the neuroscientists. Thus, he said:

> The future may teach us to exercise a direct influence, by means of particular chemical substances, upon the amounts of energy and their distribution in the apparatus of the mind. It may be that there are other undreamed-of possibilities of therapy. But for the moment we have nothing better at our disposal than the technique of psychoanalysis, and for that reason, in spite of its limitations, it is not to be despised [Freud, 1949, p. 79].

This work was supported in part by National Institute of Mental Health Grants MH 10315 and MH 13579.

References

The American Heritage Dictionary of the English Language. Houghton Mifflin Co., New York, 1973.

Andersen, H.C.: The emperor's new clothes. In Andersen's Fairy Tales, trans. by E.V. Lucas and H.B. Paull, pp. 263-268, Grosset & Dunlap, New York, 1945.

Arieti, S.: American Handbook of Psychiatry, 2nd ed., Basic Books, New York, 1974.

Bechterewa, N.P.: Physiologic und Pathophysiologic der tiefen Hirnstrukturen des Menschen, VEB Verlag Volk und Gesundheit, Berlin, 1969. (Translated into German from the Russian publication of the Academy of Medical Sciences of the USSR, 1967).

Beck, A.T.: Depression: Causes and Treatment. University of Pennsylvania Press, Philadelphia, 1967.

Bentham, J.: An introduction to the principles of morals and legislation. In The English Philosophers from Bacon to Mill, ed. by E.A. Burtt, pp. 791-852, Modern Library, New York, 1939.

Bishop, M.P., Elder, S.T. and Heath, R.G.: Intracranial self-stimulation in man. Science 140: 394-396, 1963.

Bleuler, E.: Dementia Praecox or the Group of Schizophrenias. International Universities Press, New York, 1950.

Brazier, M.A.B.: Stimulation of the hippocampus in man using implanted electrodes. In Brain Function, vol. II, pp. 299-308, University of California Press, Los Angeles, 1964.

Cannon, W.B.: The Wisdom of the Body. W.W. Norton & Co., New York, 1939.

Cannon, W.B.: Bodily Changes in Pain, Fear, Hunger, and Rage. 2nd ed., Charles T. Branford, Boston, 1953.

Carlsson, A. and Lindqvist, M.: Effect of chlorpromazine or haloperidol on the formation of 3-methoxytramine and normetanephrine in mouse brain. Acta Pharmacol. Toxicol. 20: 140-144, 1963.

Darwin, C.: On the Origin of Species. reprint of 1st ed., Watts & Co., London, 1950.

Darwin, C.: Expression of the Emotions in Man and Animal. The Philosophical Library, New York, 1955.

Delgado, J.M.R., Roberts, W.W. and Miller, N.E.: Learning motivated by electrical stimulation of the brain. Amer. J. Physiol. 179: 587, 1954.

Freedman, A.M. and Kaplan, H.I.: Comprehensive Textbook of Psychiatry. Williams & Wilkins Co., Baltimore, 1967.

Freud, S.: An Outline of Psychoanalysis. W.W. Norton & Co., New York, 1949.

Gunne, L.M.: Brain catecholamines in the rage response evoked by intracerebral stimulation and ablation. In Aggressive Behavior, ed. by A. Garattini and E.B. Sigg, pp. 238-242, John Wiley & Sons, New York, 1969.

Heath, R.G.: Electrical self-stimulation of the brain in man. Amer. J. Psychiat. 120: 571-577, 1963.

Heath, R.G.: Pleasure response of human subjects to direct stimulation of the brain: Physiologic and psychodynamic consideration. In The Role of Pleasure in Behavior, pp. 219-243, Hoeber Medical Division, Harper & Row, New York, 1964.

Heath, R.G.: Pleasure and brain activity in man. J. Nerv. Ment. Dis. 154: 3-18, 1972.

Heath, R.G., John, S.B. and Fontana, C.J.: The pleasure response: Studies by stereotaxic technics in patients. In Computers and Electronic Devices in Psychiatry, ed. by N. Kline and E. Laska, pp. 178-189, Grune & Stratton, New York, 1968.

Heath, R.G. and Mickle, W.A.: Evaluations of seven years' experience with depth electrode studies in human patients. In Electrical Studies on the Unanesthetized Brain, ed. by

E.R. Ramey and D.S. O'Doherty, pp. 214-242, Hoeber Medical Division, Harper & Row, New York, 1960.

Heston, L.L.: The genetics of schizophrenic and schizoid disease. Science 167: 249, 1970.

Jackson, J.H.: On some implications of dissolution of the nervous system. In Selected Writings of John Hughlings Jackson, ed. by J. Taylor, vol. 2, pp. 29-44, Basic Books, New York, 1958.

Jameson, J. and Klein, H.: Sandor Rado, M.D. Dr. Pol. Sci. A brief biography. In Adaptational Psychodynamics: Motivation and Control, by S. Rado, pp. ix-xiv, Science House, New York, 1969.

Kallman, F.J.: The Genetics of Schizophrenia. J.J. Augustin, New York, 1938.

Kolb, L.C.: Noyes' Modern Clinical Psychiatry. 7th ed., W.B. Saunders Co., Philadelphia, 1968.

Leibowitz, S.F.: Adrenergic receptor mechanisms in eating and drinking. In The Neurosciences, ed. by F.O. Schmitt and F.G. Worden, pp. 713-719, M.I.T. Press, Cambridge, Mass. 1974.

Matthysse, S.: Antipsychotic drug actions: A clue to the neuropathology of schizophrenia? Fed. Proc. 32: 200-205, 1973.

Meehl, P.E.: Schizotaxia, schizotypy, schizophrenia. Amer. Psychol. 17: 827-838, 1962.

Olds, J. and Milner, P.: Positive reinforcement produced by electrical stimulation of septal area and other regions. J. Comp. Physiol. Psychol. 47: 419, 1954.

The Oxford English Dictionary. Clarendon Press, Oxford, 1961.

Rado, S.: Graduate residency training in psychoanalytic medicine. Amer. J. Psychiat. 105: 111-115, 1948.

Rado, S.: Dynamics and classification of disordered behavior. Amer. J. Psychiat. 110: 406-416, 1953.

Rado, S.: Adaptational psychodynamics: A basic science. In Changing Concepts of Psychoanalytic Medicine, ed. by S. Rado and G.E. Daniels, pp. 15-30, Grune & Stratton, New York, 1956.

Rado, S.: Psychoanalytic education: Lessons of the past and responsibilities of the future. In Psychoanalysis of Behavior, Collected Papers 1956-1961, vol. 2, pp. 152-162, Grune & Stratton, New York, 1962.

Rado, S.: Hedonic self-regulation of the organism. In The Role of Pleasure in Behavior, ed. by R.G. Heath, pp. 257-264, Hoeber Medical Division, Harper & Row, New York, 1964.

Rado, S., Buchenholz, B., Dunton, H., Karlen, S.H. and Senescu, R.: Schizotypal organization. A preliminary report on a clinical study of schizophrenia. In Changing Concepts of Psychoanalytic Medicine, ed. by S. Rado and G.E. Daniels, pp. 225-235, Grune & Stratton, New York, 1956.

Reis, D.J., Miura, M., Weinbren, M. and Gunne, L.M.: Brain catecholamines: Relation to defense reaction evoked by acute brain stem transection in cat. Science 156: 1768, 1967.

Russell, B.: A History of Western Philosophy. Simon & Schuster, New York, 1945.

Schildkraut, J.J.: The catecholamine hypothesis of affective disorders: A review of supporting evidence. Amer. J. Psychiat. 122: 509-522, 1965.

Schildkraut, J.J., Gordon, E.K. and Durell, J.: Catecholamine metabolism in affective disorders: I. Normetanephrine and VMA excretion in depressed patients treated with imipramine. J. Psychiat. Res. 3: 213-228, 1965.

Schildkraut, J.J. and Kety, S.S.: Biogenic amines and emotion. Science 156: 21-30, 1967.

Sem-Jacobsen, C.W.: Depth-Electrographic Stimulation of the Human Brain and Behavior. Charles C. Thomas, Springfield, Ill., 1968.

Sem-Jacobsen, C.W. and Torkildsen, A.: Depth recording and electrical stimulation in the human brain. In Electrical Studies on the Unanesthetized Brain, ed. by E.R. Ramey and D.S. O'Doherty, pp. 275-287, Hoeber Medical Division, Harper & Row, New York, 1960.

Snyder, S.H.: Catecholamines as mediators of drug effects in schizophrenia. In The Neurosciences, ed. by F.O. Schmitt and F.G. Worden, pp. 721-732, M.I.T. Press, Cambridge, Mass., 1974.

Stein, L.: Neurochemistry of reward and punishment: Some implications for the etiology of schizophrenia. J. Psychiat. Res. 8: 345-361, 1971.

Stein, L. and Wise, C.D.: Possible etiology of schizophrenia: Progressive damage to the noradrenergic reward system by 6-hydroxydopamine. Science 171: 1032-1036, 1971.

Stein, L., Wise, C.D. and Berger, B.D.: Noradrenergic reward mechanisms, recovery of function, and schizophrenia. In The Chemistry of Mood, Motivation, and Memory, ed. by J.L. McGaugh, pp. 81-103, Plenum Press, New York, 1972.

Valenstein, E.S.: Brain Control. A Critical Examination of Brain Stimulation and Psychosurgery. John Wiley & Sons, New York, 1973.

Watson, J.B.: Psychology as the behaviorist views it. Psychol. Rev. 20: 158-177, 1913.

Webster's Third New International Dictionary. G. & C. Merriam Co., Springfield, Mass., 1968.

Wise, C.D. and Stein, L.: Dopamine-β-hydroxylase deficits in the brains of schizophrenic patients. Science 181: 344-347, 1973.

Wise, C.D. and Stein, L.: Evidence of a central noradrenergic deficit in schizophrenia. In Neurotransmitter Balances Regulating Behavior, ed. and published by E.F. Domino and J.M. Davis, pp. 99-123, Ann Arbor, Michigan, 1975.

Neurotransmitter Balances Regulating Behavior,
edited and published by E.F. Domino and
J.M. Davis, Ann Arbor, © 1975

PSYCHOANALYTIC CONCEPTS AND BRAIN STIMULATION: FURTHER CONSIDERATIONS OF RELEVANCE

Dennis D. Kelly
New York State Psychiatric Institute
and
Columbia University
New York, New York

Murray Glusman (1975) raises several scholarly issues critical to the biochemical model of schizophrenia put forward by Stein and Wise (1971). Their model proposes that, if the bizarre behaviors of the schizophrenic can be characterized as a unitary deficiency in pleasure regulation or goal directed behavior, that is, as fundamentally an anhedonic syndrome, then its etiology might be related to synaptic damage in the brain's noradrenergic reward system. In turn, the neuropathology is presumed to result from the degenerative activities of an endogenously manufactured toxin, 6-hydroxydopamine, the formation of the latter triggered by either a stress-induced or gene-related irregularity in norepinephrine metabolism (Stein, 1971; Stein and Wise, 1971, 1972). In evaluating this proposal, Glusman has questioned whether anhedonia represents an adequate, or even historically accurate, characterization of schizophrenia, indeed whether anhedonia is even a consistent symptom of schizophrenia. It more commonly appears in the diagnosis of depression. Glusman also raised the issue as to whether the probable behavioral role mediated by the neural reward and punishment systems cited by Stein and Wise corresponds in any meaningful way with the psychoanalytic construct of hedonic self-regulation upon which Stein and Wise lean heavily in attempting to establish the relevance of their neurochemical work to the broader problem of schizophrenia. The noradrenergic reward pathways singled out in the model have been empirically defined with operational simplicity through self-stimulation experiments in mute animals; the connecting psychoanalytic concept is a speculation of Sandor Rado.

To clarify Rado's notions on pleasure and anhedonia as they might relate to psychopathology, Glusman has offered an interesting historical sketch of Rado's roots in the utilitarian line of philosophers deriving from Jeremy Bentham and John Stuart Mill. It might prove equally instructive to complete this historical perspective by extending it here to reinforcement theory, for it is from the latter tradition that the techniques and concepts sprang, such as the law of effect, that made possible the empirical charting of the "pleasure" pathways of the brain by Olds and the eventual analysis of their neurochemistry by Stein and Wise. This perspective may reveal that in contemporary usage the notions of reward and reinforcement in experimental psychology differ substantially from Rado's psychodynamic views of pleasure and hedonic self-regulation. The two concepts stem from distinctly different historical lines. They are also cast from very unlike theoretical propositions, and thus translation of each in terms of the other turns out to be a hazardous task, at best.

In modern form, the notion of reinforcement refers to the empirical observation that those behaviors that meet with good consequences seem to be repeated at the expense of behaviors that do not, while behaviors followed by aversive, though not necessarily only painful, consequences seldom are repeated. A consensus currently exists among experimental psychologists that this simple notion probably reflects an important law that governs much apparently voluntary behavior. In turn, the consensus seems to have its roots in an objective, Anglo-American tradition of psychologists that can be traced directly to the British animal psychologists of the late nineteenth century, notably, to C. Lloyd Morgan (1852-1936).[1] Morgan's primary research interests lay in analyzing the relation of the animal mind to that of man, and in these matters he drew heavily upon the ideas of Herbert Spencer (1820-1903), who, though better known as a proponent of "Social Darwinianism," also authored one of the first systematic, scientifically plausible theories of the learning process (Spencer, 1870). Morgan's relatively strict, conservative approach represented a strong methodological reaction - in fact, one that has endured until the present day in English-speaking circles - against the then fashionable tendency to anthropomorphize the acts of animals freely and to attribute to them human mental motives. His "law of parsimony" is still known as Lloyd's Canon and its original formulation in 1894, applied to animal psychology, read:

> In no case, may we interpret an action as the outcome of the exercise of a higher psychical faculty, if it can be interpreted as the outcome of the exercise of one which stands lower in the psychological scale [Morgan, 1894].

[1]For a more extensive history, the reader should consult Postman (1947) and the recent, very fine chapter by Wilcoxon (1969), which should also be acknowledged in the preparation of this section.

Less a momentous law than simply a rule of thumb, Morgan suggested here that we try to interpret animal behavior in the simplest possible terms.[2] And, the "lower level of functioning" toward which Morgan's word of advice directed attention was the "pleasure tropism," or the "law of effect," as it was immediately thereafter formalized by Edward Lee Thorndike (1874-1949).

Thorndike's thesis research on the puzzle box, concluded in 1898 but published along with some additional work in 1911 in Animal Intelligence, firmly established the law of effect in learning. Thorndike prepared fifteen puzzle boxes for cats, dogs, and chicks in which the animal was locked and from which it could escape by pulling a chain, nosing a bobbin, or by performing any one of as many as fifteen odd mechanical tricks. Learning curves were plotted indicating how long it took a cat to escape on the first trial, how long on the second, and so on. The gently sloping shape of the curves suggested to Thorndike that the cats learned to get out, as he put it, "by trial and error and accidental success." To this day this is known as "trial-and-error" learning, but, as Wilcoxon (1969) aptly notes, Thorndike himself was more concerned with the success. To him it was obvious that the success of a correct movement, although it resulted from the movement, in turn caused the movement to be learned. The success is the effect of the movement, and it appears to "stamp in" those movements that caused it. Indeed, Thorndike's is probably the first description of a behavioral feedback loop. Initially, Thorndike identified success with pleasure and, soon, with satisfaction. Thus:

> The law of effect is that: Of several responses made in the same situation, those which are accompanied or closely followed by satisfaction to the animal will, other things being equal, be more firmly connected to the situation, so that, when it recurs, they will be more likely to recur; those which are

[2]In current scientific circles, the law of parsimony, or Occam's razor, continues to enjoy frequent mention but less than legal status. It cannot be any more than a working hypothesis that behavior, and consequently the nervous system, should operate by the most simple conceivable set of rules. In fact, biological examples of parallel evolution would seem to have firmly established the principle that a given physiologic process, such as respiration, can evolve to varying degrees of complexity in different species, all with the same net end. A scientist's labor is to explain nature as he finds it, not as he might more elegantly or thriftily redesign it.

> accompanied or closely followed by discomfort to the animal will, other things being equal, have their connections with the situation weakened, so that, when it recurs, they will be less likely to occur. The greater the satisfaction or discomfort, the greater the strengthening or weakening of the bond [Thorndike, 1911, p. 244].

Referred to the puzzle box experiments, this descriptive law seemed to fit Thorndike's observations well. Cats began by using instinctive movements, stumbled upon success, which then "stamped in" the movement of which it was the effect.

The major difficulty subsequently encountered in generalizing the law beyond the puzzle box centered upon the definition of what was meant by a "satisfying state" of a response. For example, much later Hull (1943) was to define it as a reduction in a biological drive, an assumption that created almost as many exceptions as to its rule as members (Miller, 1963). In the meantime, Thorndike's own concept of reinforcement evolved quite broadly over the years so as to include by 1933, for instance, even "a purely symbolic satisfier, such as the anouncement of 'Right' in an experiment in learning" (Thorndike, 1933). Following the post-war trend towards strong empiricism in the study of learning, the answer as to what constitutes a rewarding satisfaction has equally often been reflected back upon the behavior that is strengthened - in an operational, if potentially circular, manner - thereby avoiding controversy over the nature of satisfaction (Meehl, 1950). Thus, Keller and Schoenfeld (1950) defined positive reinforcers as "those stimuli which strengthen responses when presented" (p. 61). In this manner, events, or stimuli, may be defined empirically as reinforcers, not in terms of any effects they might have upon the internal functions of the organism (such as reducing a tissue need), but strictly in terms of the effects they have upon the probability of a behavioral response.

Certainly the most powerful new reinforcer identified by this operational approach was the direct electrical stimulation through permanently implanted wires of various regions of the mammalian forebrain (Olds and Milner, 1954). Sites whose stimulation supported high rates of lever pressing or motivated mastery of a maze, as examples of the defining behaviors used, were defined and mapped as positively reinforcing or rewarding areas, and the pathways connecting these sites were proposed as "reward" systems (Olds and Olds, 1963; Stein, 1969). In a similar manner so called "punishment" systems have been traced using the conventional empirical criteria for defining negative reinforcers, such as the strengthening of responses that remove the intracranial stimulation (ICS) in question, suppression of responses that produce it, and so on.

This behavioral scheme for sorting out operationally equivalent brain sites imparted a rigor and economy to ICS research in the past two decades that required no additional theoretical justification. The heuristic value of the simple behavioral classifications proved enormous, and the straightforward rationale adequately supported the subsequent tide of experiments executed within the framework provided by these specific, defining behaviors. However, as the produce of this internally consistent line of research becomes extrapolated to broader problems, such as the cause of schizophrenia, it becomes important to pursue the question of whether the accumulated evidence, and its method of acquisition, support the notion of a neural "reward" pathway as such. In other words, whether there exists a system whose specific purpose is to provide reinforcement for behaviors and, hence, whose malfunction could result in an across-the-board disruption in the process by which newly adaptive behaviors are acquired. As many researchers are aware, there are a number of findings that argue against a literal acceptance of self-stimulation data as proof of a "reward" system. For one, few electrode sites ever exhibit pure rewarding, or pure punishing effects, and to the extent of such ambivalent results, the binary classification of neural systems as rewarding or punishing is itself suspect. Generally speaking, a train of even highly reinforcing, pulsed stimulations will become aversive by operational criteria if left on for a matter of seconds instead of only milliseconds (Bower and Miller, 1958; Roberts, 1958; Beer and Steiner, 1965; Cooper and Taylor, 1967; Steiner _et al_., 1969; Steiner _et al_., 1973; Ellman _et al_., 1975). This is true even at low intensities where spread of current to adjacent punishment systems is unlikely. An even more troubling parameter of the reinforcing valence of an ICS site is the degree of instrumental control over the ICS that is afforded the subject. Thus, Steiner _et al_. (1969) found that a rat will work with equal diligence to escape from the same tape-recorded pattern of ICS that it generated through its own performance the day before. In fact, this study seems to have anticipated an accelerating literature that emphasizes the importance of the subject's control over the delivery of the ICS in determining whether the net effect of a stimulation is rewarding, neutral, or even punishing (Meyers and Valenstein, 1964; Cantor and LoLordo, 1970; Cantor, 1971;

Bollinger et al., 1972; Faircloth, 1974). While it may be premature to draw strong revisionary conclusions, we ought at least to acknowledge that the reinforcing properties of those ICS sites, initially defined simply as "reward" or "pleasure" areas, are not as unmalleable as the original behavioral criteria made them appear. They may, with further behavioral study, prove as sensitive to subtle organismic factors, like self-control, as to the traditional stimulus variables, such as charge, waveform, pulse duration, site of the electrode, etc., emphasized by earlier work. As Glusman noted in support of Valenstein's (1973) scholarly review, electrical stimulation of these same sites in humans produces a wide, almost disconnected range of subjective phenomena.

So, in retrospect, the evolution of the original law of effect into the current construct of reinforcement in the behavioral sciences has importantly shaped some of our inferences concerning brain function, at least those immediately derived from self-stimulation and preference experiments. That Stein and Wise should now find these inferences forming a parallel to certain psychoanalytic concepts is an interesting development, in that the particular version of the law of effect that serviced self-stimulation research in the most recent two decades probably represents, in the broader scheme, only one particular phase in the continuing evolution of the concept of reinforcement. Indeed, the durability of reinforcement theory and the law of effect, in particular, must in part be attributed to its continual amendment and sharpening. Current reformulations which emphasize the evolutionary analogy (reinforcement is seen as selecting among already occurring behaviors in a manner similar to natural biological selection among phenotypes) and a "contingency" versus "contiguity" based process of reinforcement bear scant resemblance to either Thorndike's original precept or to the austere, operational version employed in self-stimulation research (Perkins, 1968; Gilbert, 1970, 1972; Herrnstein, 1970; Seligman, 1970; Staddon and Simmelhag, 1971; Staddon, 1972, 1973; Baum, 1973). It is hard to avoid the impression that reinforcement theory, as considered here, and Rado's notions, as sketched by Glusman, are not unlike two vessels which, having sailed from different ports and likely headed on different courses, were now passing in mid-voyage with a proximity that is, at best, difficult to judge.

As a final and more positive note, it is true that in the past the behavioristic and psychoanalytic traditions have each taken positions and struck attitudes that the other found inimical, particularly concerning the status of subjective phenomena in an evolving science of behavior. Glusman is undoubtedly correct in projecting Sandor Rado's probable dismay with the strict, anti-introspectionist credo expressed by the young Watson. On the other hand, it is interesting that early leaders, indeed, the founders, of both movements held overlapping aspirations for the future explanation of their respective phenomena by neurobiologic research. John Broadus Watson always felt, dating from his early associations with Jennings and Adolph Meyer at Johns Hopkins, that the basis of habit formation might eventually be discovered in physiological terms, but only in the distant future:

> Fortunately, we can continue our work in behavior without awaiting the true explanation of these biological phenomena couched in physiochemical terms [Watson, 1930, p. 210].

In the very same year, Sigmund Freud wrote in a letter to Marie Bonaparte:

> We know that the mechanisms of the psychoses are in essence no different from those of the neuroses, but we do not have at our disposal the quantitative stimulation necessary for changing them. The hope of the future here lies in organic chemistry or the access to it through endocrinology. This future is still far distant, but one should study analytically every case of psychosis because this knowledge will one day guide the chemical therapy [Jones, 1957, p. 449].

References

Baum, W.M.: The correlation-based law of effect. J. Exp. Anal. Behav. 20: 137-153, 1973.

Beer, B. and Steiner, S.S.: An analysis of the ambivalent properties of electrical brain stimulation. Paper presented at the meeting of the Psychonomic Society, Chicago, October, 1965.

Bollinger, S.F., Faircloth, K. and Doering, R.M.: The instrumental response and hypothalamic stimulus-bound drinking. Physiol. Behav. 8: 377-381, 1972.

Bower, G.H. and Miller, N.E.: Rewarding and punishing effects from stimulating the same place in the rat's brain. J. Comp. Physiol. Psychol. 51: 669-674, 1958.

Cantor, M.B.: Signaled reinforcing brain stimulation facilitates operant behavior under schedules of intermittent reinforcement. Science 174: 610-613, 1971.

Cantor, M.B. and LoLordo, V.: Rats prefer signaled reinforcing brain stimulation to unsignaled EBS. J. Comp. Physiol. Psych. 71: 183-191, 1970.

Cantor, M.B. and LoLordo, V.: Reward value of brain stimulation is inversely related to uncertainty about its onset. J. Comp. Physiol. Psych. 79: 259-270, 1972.

Cooper, R.M. and Taylor, L.H.: Thalamic reticular system and central grey: Self-stimulation. Science 156: 102-103, 1967.

Ellman, S.J., Ackermann, R.F., Bodnar, R., Jackler, F. and Steiner, S.S.: Comparison of behaviors elicited by electrical brain stimulation in dorsal brain stem and hypothalamus of rats. J. Comp. Physiol. Psychol. 88: 816-828, 1975.

Faircloth, K.: The importance of subject control in reinforcing brain stimulation. Learn. Motivat. 5: 16-23, 1974.

Gilbert, R.M.: Psychology and biology. Canadian Psychologists 11: 221-238, 1970.

Gilbert, R.M.: Variation and selection of behavior. In Reinforcement: Behavioral Analyses, ed. by R.M. Gilbert and J.R. Millenson, pp. 263-276, Academic Press, New York, 1972.

Glusman, M.: Psychoanalytic concepts and brain stimulation: A consideration of relevance. In Neurotransmitter Balances Regulating Behavior, ed. and published by E.F. Domino and J.M. Davis, pp. 1-23, Ann Arbor, Michigan, 1975.

Herrnstein, R.J.: On the law of effect. J. Exp. Anal. Behav. 13: 243-266, 1970.

Hull, C.L.: Principles of Behavior, Appleton, New York, 1943.

Jones, E.: The Life and Work of Sigmund Freud, Vol. 3, Basic Books, New York, 1957.

Keller, F.S. and Schoenfeld, W.N.: Principles of Psychology, Appleton-Century-Crofts, New York, 1950.

Meehl, P.E.: On the circularity of the law of effect. Psychol. Bull. 47: 42-75, 1950.

Meyers, W.J. and Valenstein, E.S.: Animal preference for method of obtaining reinforcing brain stimulation. J. Comp. Physiol. Psychol. 57: 47-51, 1964.

Miller, N.E.: Some reflections on the law of effect produce a new alternative to drive reduction. In Nebraska Symposium on Motivation, ed. by M.R. Jones, pp. 65-112, University of Nebraska, Lincoln, 1963.

Morgan, C.L.: Introduction to Comparative Psychology, W. Scott, London, 1894.

Olds, J. and Milner, P.: Positive reinforcement produced by electrical stimulation of septal area and other regions of the rat brain. J. Comp. Physiol. Psychol. 47: 419-427, 1954.

Olds, J. and Olds, M.E.: Approach-avoidance analysis of rat diencephalon. J. Comp. Neurol. 120: 259-295, 1963.

Perkins, C.C.: An analysis of the concept of reinforcement. Psychol. Rev. 75: 155-172, 1968.

Postman, L.: The history and present status of the law of effect. Psychol. Bull. 44: 489-563, 1947.

Roberts, W.W.: Both rewarding and punishing effects from stimulation of posterior hypothalamus of cat with same electrode at same intensity. J. Comp. Physiol. Psychol. 51: 400-407, 1958.

Seligman, M.E.P.: On the generality of the laws of learning. Psychol. Rev. 77: 406-418, 1970.

Spencer, H.: The Principles of Psychology, Vol. 1 (2nd Ed.), Appleton, New York, 1870.

Staddon, J.E.R.: Temporal control and the theory of reinforcement schedules. In Reinforcement: Behavioral Analyses, ed. by R.M. Gilbert and J. Millenson, pp. 212-262, Academic Press, New York, 1972.

Staddon, J.E.R.: On the notion of cause, with applications to behaviorism. Behaviorism 1: 25-63, 1973.

Staddon, J.E.R. and Simmelhag, V.: The "superstition" experiment: A re-examination of its implications for the principles of adaptive behavior. Psychol. Rev. 78: 3-43, 1971.

Stein, L.: Chemistry of purposive behavior. In Reinforcement and Behavior, ed. by J. Tapp, pp. 238-355, Academic Press, New York, 1969.

Stein, L.: Neurochemistry of reward and punishment: Some implications for the etiology of schizophrenia. J. Psychiat. Res. 8: 345-361, 1971.

Stein, L. and Wise, C.D.: Possible etiology of schizophrenia: Progressive damage to the noradrenergic reward system by 6-hydroxydopamine. Science 171: 1032-1036, 1971.

Stein, L. and Wise, C.D.: Possible etiology of schizophrenia: Progressive damage to the noradrenergic reward system by endogenous 6-hydroxydopamine. Neurotransmitters, Research Publ. Assoc. Research Nerv. Ment. Disease 50: 298-311, 1972.

Steiner, S.S., Beer, B. and Schaffer, M.: Escape from self-produced rates of brain stimulation. Science 163: 90-91, 1969.

Steiner, S.S., Bodnar, R.J., Ackermann, R.F. and Ellman, S.J.: Escape from rewarding brain stimulation of dorsal brainstem and hypothalamus. Physiol. Behav. 177: 589-591, 1973.

Thorndike, E.L.: Animal Intelligence, Macmillan, New York, 1911. (Reprinted edition available from Haefner Publ. Co., 1970).

Thorndike, E.L.: A theory of the action of the after-effects of a connection upon it. Psychol. Rev. 40: 434-439, 1933.

Valenstein, E.S.: Brain Control: A Critical Examination of Brain Stimulation and Psychosurgery, John Wiley & Sons, New York, 1973.

Watson, J.B.: Behaviorism. (Rev. Ed.) Norton, New York, 1930.

Wilcoxon, H.C.: Historical introduction to the problem of reinforcement. In Reinforcement and Behavior, ed. by J. Tapp, pp. 1-46, Academic Press, New York, 1969.

Neurotransmitter Balances Regulating Behavior,
edited and published by E.F. Domino and
J.M. Davis, Ann Arbor, © 1975

RELATIONSHIP OF DOPAMINE NEURAL SYSTEMS TO THE MAINTENANCE OF SELF-STIMULATION

George R. Breese and Barrett R. Cooper
Departments of Psychiatry and Pharmacology
Biological Sciences Research Center of
The Child Development Institute
University of North Carolina
School of Medicine
Chapel Hill, North Carolina

In 1954, Olds and Milner reported that animals would press a bar to obtain an electrical stimulus through electrodes implanted in certain regions of brain. Olds (1958) later suggested that in stimulating these brain structures the animal was activating a reward system. This latter view has been particularly attractive to investigators who have been interested in relating drives and motivation to anatomical substrates (Deutsch and Howarth, 1963; Miller, 1963; Stein, 1968). Evidence that self-stimulation was most readily obtained from electrodes implanted in the lateral hypothalamus (Olds, 1962; Valenstein, 1966) and the demonstration that the medial forebrain bundle, coursing through the lateral hypothalamic area, contained axons of biogenic amine neurons (Fuxe, 1965; Ungerstedt, 1971; Fuxe and Johnson, 1974) suggested that intracranial electrical self-stimulation might be related to activation of a monoamine pathway.

Since many agents which alter self-stimulation behavior have an effect on central adrenergic mechanisms, there has been much speculation concerning the relationship of central catecholamine neural pathways to the anatomical substrate of self-stimulation and "reward" (Poschel and Ninteman, 1963; Stein, 1964, 1967, 1968; Crow, 1972). Several studies have demonstrated that compounds believed to increase central adrenergic tone, such as monoamine oxidase inhibitors (Poschel and Ninteman, 1964; Poschel, 1969), *d*-amphetamine (Stein, 1964, 1967; Poschel and Ninteman, 1966; Stein and Wise, 1973), and cocaine (Crow, 1970), have been found to increase self-stimulation, whereas agents which reduce central adrenergic tone such as reserpine (Stein, 1962), chlorpromazine (Olds and Travis, 1960; Stein, 1962) or α-methyltyrosine (Gibson *et al.*, 1970; Black and Cooper, 1970) all reduced self-stimulation behavior.

Effect of intracisternally-administered 6-hydroxydopamine on self-stimulation. Since 6-hydroxydopamine was found to reduce norepinephrine and dopamine content in brain (Uretsky and Iversen, 1970; Breese and Traylor, 1970, 1971), treatment with this compound provided an additional method by which to examine the role of catecholamine neural systems in the maintenance of this task. Animals implanted with electrodes aimed at the lateral hypothalamus were treated intracisternally with 6-hydroxydopamine after being trained to press a bar for self-stimulation (Breese *et al.*, 1971). As shown in figure 1, there was an acute reduction of bar pressing with performance recovering within a few days to 50 to 60 percent of control. Responding remained

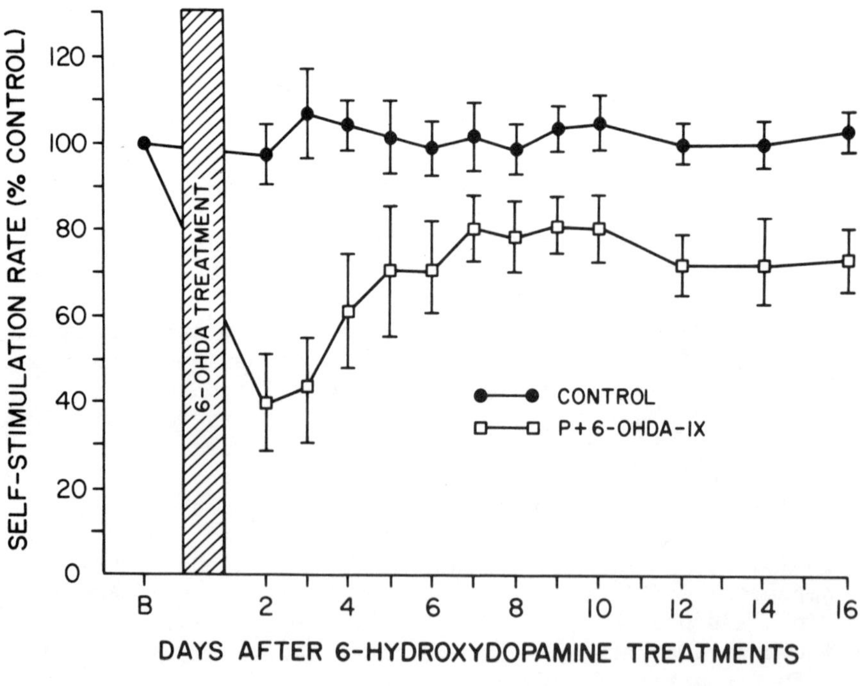

Fig. 1. Effect of 6-hydroxydopamine (P + 6-OHDA-1X) on lateral hypothalamic self-stimulation. Animals received 200 μg 6-OHDA intracisternally 30 min after pargyline (Breese *et al.*, 1971 and Cooper *et al.*, 1974).

significantly reduced 35 days after treatment, suggesting that the deficit was permanent (Breese *et al*., 1971). A second injection of 6-hydroxydopamine virtually eliminated self-stimulation responding (Breese *et al*., 1971). At about the same time, these results were confirmed by Stein and Wise (1971), providing additional support for the importance of catecholamine-containing fibers in the maintenance of self-stimulation of the brain.

Effect of preferential destruction of noradrenergic and dopaminergic neural pathways on self-stimulation. While the above studies did not provide information concerning the importance of individual catecholamine neural systems, additional studies showing that the depression of self-stimulation produced by the dopamine-β-hydroxylase inhibitor, disulfiram, was reversed by intracerebral injections of norepinephrine (Wise and Stein, 1969) resulted in the suggestion that self-stimulation behavior was maintained by a noradrenergic neural system. Additional support for this hypothesis came with the observation that self-stimulation could be obtained from placements in the norepinephrine cell bodies of the locus coeruleus (Crow *et al*., 1972; Ritter and Stein, 1973). Furthermore, electrical stimulation of rewarding sites in brain has been found to increase the efflux of radioactivity after administration of H^3-norepinephrine, indicating that norepinephrine is released during self-stimulation behavior (Stein and Wise, 1969).

Recently, however, evidence has accumulated which suggests that self-stimulation is not strictly a noradrenergic phenomenon. The relationship of the action of disulfiram to an effect on noradrenergic fibers to decrease self-stimulation (e.g., Wise and Stein, 1969) has been challenged by Roll (1970) who argued that the effects of this drug were related to a more general disruption of arousal. Furthermore, the more recently developed dopamine-β-hydroxylase inhibitors, such as FLA-63, are not reported to have a significant depressant effect on self-stimulation behavior (Lippa *et al*., 1973).

In addition to evidence that implicated noradrenergic fibers, new evidence has suggested that dopamine neural systems in brain may be important to the maintenance of self-stimulation. Involvement of dopaminergic fibers in this behavior is based on findings that high rates of self-stimulation occur from electrodes placed in the substantia nigra and that an increased rate of dopamine turnover accompanies rewarding stimulation of such sites (Crow, 1972; Arbuthnott *et al*., 1970). Evidence also exists that the postulated dopamine receptor blocking compound, haloperidol, decreases self-stimulation of the lateral hypothalamus

(Wauquier and Niemegeers, 1972; Lippa *et al.*, 1973), while phentolamine, a noradrenergic blocking agent, does not (Lippa *et al.*, 1973). Similar results have also been re-reported following pimozide (Wauquier and Niemegeers, 1972; Liebman and Butcher, 1973). Finally, Phillips and Fibiger (1973) have related the different biochemical effects of *d*- and *l*-amphetamine with regard to norepinephrine or dopamine uptake into synaptosomes (e.g., Taylor and Snyder, 1970, 1971) to differential effects on self-stimulation obtained from noradrenergic or dopaminergic sites in brain.

From this discussion, it should be clear that a distinction between a possible role for norepinephrine or dopamine-containing fibers in the maintenance of self-stimulation has become one of the central questions with regard to a "catecholamine hypothesis of self-stimulation." Recently, methods have been developed to destroy norepinephrine or dopamine-containing fibers in brain (Breese and Traylor, 1971) and these have been used to examine the role of central sympathetic neural systems in self-stimulation (Breese *et al.*, 1973; Cooper *et al.*, 1974; Breese *et al.*, 1974). Since rates of intracranial self-stimulation have been found to be highest from the electrodes placed in the lateral hypothalamus, this was the first site chosen for investigation. Results of this study are summarized in figure 2. While the treatment which preferentially reduced brain dopamine with little effect on noradrenergic fibers (DA ↓) (Breese and Traylor, 1971) caused an acute depression of responding, rates of self-stimulation returned to a level which did not differ significantly from control by 5 days after injection.

Previous work has shown that rats which had recovered behaviorally from the initial depression produced by 6-hydroxydopamine displayed an enhanced sensitivity to doses of α-methyltyrosine which did not affect responding in control animals (Cooper *et al.*, 1972, 1973; Breese *et al.*, 1973). Since chronic deficits in self-stimulation did not occur in the rats treated with 6-hydroxydopamine, α-methyltyrosine was administered to each of the groups and its effects on self-stimulation determined (Breese *et al.*, 1973, 1974; Cooper *et al.*, 1974). As shown in figure 3, when α-methyltyrosine was administered to rats in which both brain catecholamines were reduced or to rats which had just brain dopamine preferentially destroyed (DA ↓) self-stimulation behavior was significantly reduced, whereas bar press responding for self-stimulation remained unaffected in control rats and rats treated to destroy noradrenergic fibers in brain.

Strong evidence has previously been provided to indicate

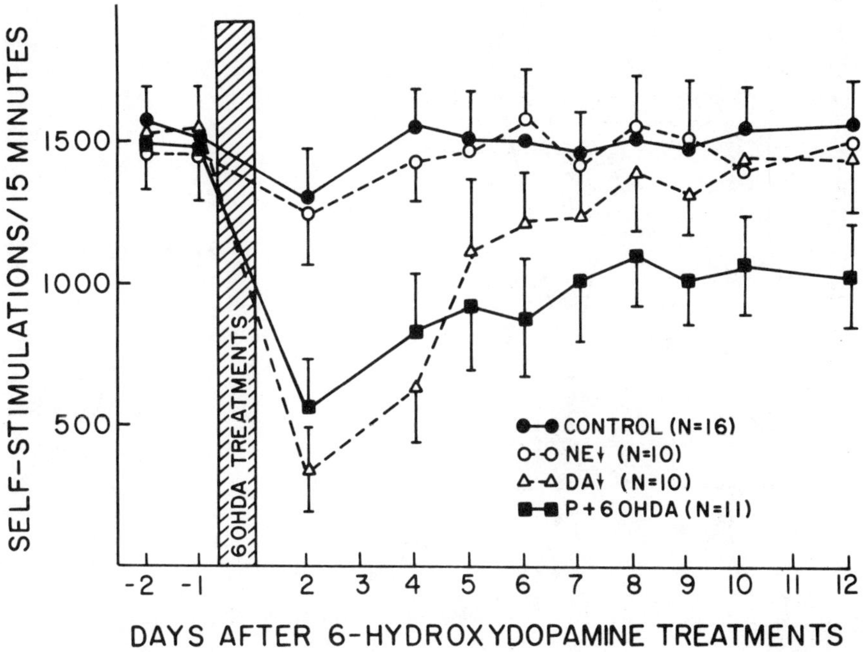

Fig. 2. Effect of norepinephrine, dopamine or catecholamine destruction with 6-hydroxydopamine on lateral hypothalamic self-stimulation. NE↓ refers to rats treated with 3 x 25 μg 6-OHDA and DA↓ refers to rats that received desipramine (25 mg/kg) 60 min before receiving 6-OHDA (200 μg). The P+6-OHDA treatment is the same as P+6-OHDA-IX in Fig. 1 (see Breese and Traylor, 1971; Cooper et al., 1973, 1974).

a role of norepinephrine in self-stimulation behavior (Stein, 1968; Crow, 1972). It was of interest, therefore, to determine if an additional depletion of brain norepinephrine with the dopamine-β-hydroxylase inhibitor (U-14,624)

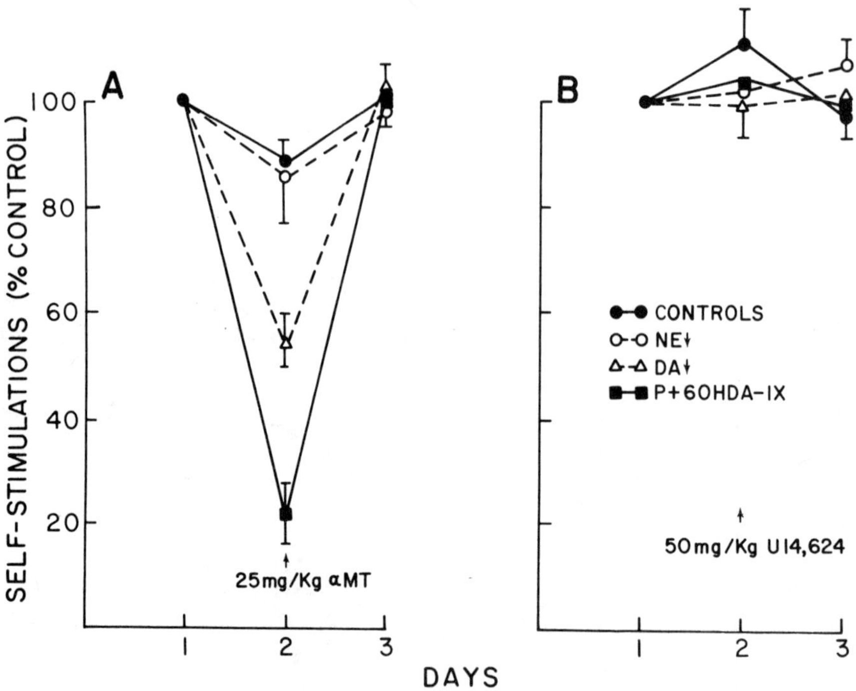

Fig. 3. Effects of α-methyltyrosine (α-MT) or U-14,624 on self-stimulation responding in rats treated with 6-hydroxydopamine. Doses of α-MT and U-14,624 were administered 4 and 6 hr, respectively, before behavioral testing (see Breese et al., 1973, 1974; Cooper et al., 1974).

would provide deficits in rats treated intracisternally with 6-hydroxydopamine which could be correlated with the concentration of norepinephrine remaining in brain. When self-stimulating animals were examined 6 hours after treatment with 50 mg/kg of U-14,624, there were no significant differences between any of the 6-hydroxydopamine treatment groups (figure 3B). It was also observed that FLA-63 did not reduce self-stimulation responding of animals depleted of norepinephrine (unpublished data). Table 1 shows that levels of norepinephrine in brain were reduced by an

Table 1

Effect of α-Methyltyrosine and U-14,624 on Brain Catecholamine Content After Various 6-Hydroxydopamine Treatments

Treatment	Untreated Rats		α-Methyltyrosine		U-14,624	
	NE	DA	NE	DA	NE	DA
Control	425 ± 29	573 ± 28	259 ± 30*	315 ± 40*	114 ± 25*	670 ± 108
NE ↓	165 ± 17	492 ± 40	89 ± 4*	303 ± 34*	34 ± 8*	521 ± 63
DA ↓	369 ± 29	171 ± 28	221 ± 17*	103 ± 23*	113 ± 13*	149 ± 17
P + 6-OHDA	110 ± 13	126 ± 11	46 ± 16*	40 ± 17*	20 ± 4*	143 ± 45

All values for norepinephrine (NE) and dopamine (DA) are expressed as mμg/g. Rats were treated with α-methyltyrosine (25 mg/kg) or U-14,624 (50 mg/kg) as described in figure 3.
*P <.01 when compared with control rats of the same control or 6-hydroxydopamine treatment condition.

additional 70 percent in all 6-hydroxydopamine treatment groups given U-14,624. Of particular note was the fact that only about 8 percent of the norepinephrine remained in brain of rats previously treated to deplete this amine (NE ↓). The concentration of dopamine in brain following this treatment was not significantly affected (Table 1).

Role of catecholamine-fibers in the effects of amphetamine on self-stimulation. It is well known that d-amphetamine facilitates motor activity, an effect proposed to be related to release of central catecholamines (Weissman et al., 1966; Hanson, 1966). Although earlier work had suggested that d-amphetamine stimulated motor activity was related to indirect release of norepinephrine in brain (Randrup and Scheel-Krüger, 1966), more recent evidence has suggested that indirect release of dopamine is responsible for the locomotor stimulation produced by d-amphetamine (Hollister et al., 1974). d-Amphetamine has also been reported to facilitate electrical self-stimulation of brain (Stein, 1964; Crow, 1969), an action of d-amphetamine which also has been proposed to be related to an indirect release of brain norepinephrine (Stein, 1964; Stein and Wise, 1973).

In order to obtain further information concerning the neurochemical basis of self-stimulation, the possible relationship of the stimulant actions of d-amphetamine on self-stimulation to intact catecholamine neural systems was examined in rats in which either brain norepinephrine or dopamine was preferentially reduced (Cooper et al., 1974). In this study, current intensity was adjusted to a level that just maintained responding. Animals were then treated with 0.25 mg/kg of d-amphetamine sulfate. Figure 4 shows that bar pressing rates of control animals was markedly enhanced by this amphetamine treatment. Responding of animals in which brain norepinephrine was preferentially reduced (NE ↓) was not significantly different from that observed in the control group. However, responding of rats in which brain dopamine was preferentially reduced (DA ↓) remained significantly below that of the other groups. This included a reduction in the peak effect 30 min after d-amphetamine as well as in the total responses during the 75 min experimental period. In a second experiment, control rats and animals preferentially depleted of norepinephrine (NE ↓) were treated with U-14,624 six hr prior to amphetamine (0.25 mg/kg). Depletion of norepinephrine in this manner also failed to significantly alter the increased responding produced by d-amphetamine treatment (Cooper et al., 1974).

Since the results of the preceding experiments suggested

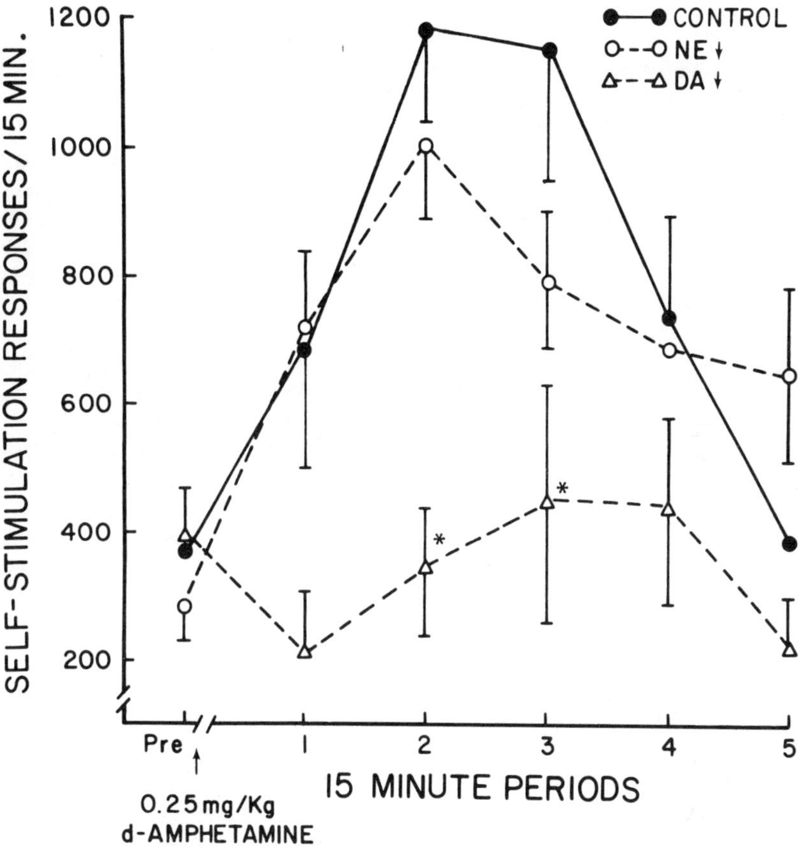

Fig. 4. Effects of d-amphetamine on lateral hypothalamic self-stimulation in rats in which brain norepinephrine (NE ↓) or brain dopamine (DA ↓) have been preferentially reduced. A threshold current level which just maintained responding was determined for each rat prior to treatment with d-amphetamine sulfate. **P < .05 when compared with control.

that intact dopaminergic neural function was required for the effects of amphetamine on self-stimulation obtained from the lateral hypothalamus, confirmation of this possibility was sought using another approach. The ability of α-methyltyrosine, but not reserpine to block the locomotor stimulant effects of d-amphetamine has been used to argue for the importance of newly synthesized catecholamines in the actions of this compound (Hanson, 1966). Therefore, it was subsequently reasoned that rats could be treated with reserpine and then given α-methyltyrosine to inhibit synthesis of catecholamines or given U-14,624 to inhibit synthesis of just norepinephrine before determining the response to d-amphetamine (Cooper *et al.*, 1974). When these animals were injected with 1 mg/kg d-amphetamine sulfate, rats that received only reserpine showed a marked increase in responding (figure 5). Similar to this observation, rats that received reserpine followed 24 hr later with the U-14,624 treatment also increased their self-stimulation rates. Animals treated with reserpine followed 24 hr later by α-methyltyrosine failed to respond to d-amphetamine treatment (figure 5).

Investigations of self-stimulation from the locus coeruleus. While providing convincing evidence that dopaminergic neural systems in brain have an important function in the maintenance of self-stimulation from the lateral hypothalamus, the data thus far described did not indicate a role for norepinephrine. Since self-stimulation occurs from electrode placements in areas containing cell bodies and pathways of the dorsal noradrenergic neural system (Crow, 1972), it was felt that the precise relationship of norepinephrine-containing neurons to self-stimulation required further investigation. In this phase of our research, animals were implanted in the locus coeruleus and the effects of a dopamine-β-hydroxylase inhibitor on self-stimulation responding examined. In addition, the effects of d-amphetamine on locus coeruleus self-stimulation in reserpinized rats in the presence and absence of U-14,624 or α-methyltyrosine was assessed (Cooper *et al.*, 1974).

As shown in table 2, treatment with U-14,624 did not affect self-stimulation responding from electrodes aimed at the locus coeruleus, while treatment with α-methyltyrosine produced a reduction in responding. This was particularly surprising, since α-methyltyrosine reduced norepinephrine content by only 50 percent whereas U-14,624 reduced norepinephrine by 73 percent. These data seemed to provide evidence that self-stimulation from the locus coeruleus was also dependent upon intact dopaminergic systems.

In additional experiments to understand the role of catecholamines in the maintenance of self-stimulation, animals with locus coeruleus electrode placements were treated with reserpine (Cooper *et al.*, 1974). As in experiments described earlier, animals were treated with α-methyltyrosine or U-14,624 and then given d-amphetamine. As shown in table 3, α-methyltyrosine blocked the stimulation produced by d-amphetamine while treatment with U-14,624 did not. Thus, these preliminary studies of the psychopharmacology of locus coeruleus self-stimulation also

Table 2

Effect of α-Methyltyrosine and U-14,624 on Locus Coeruleus

Self-Stimulation and Brain Catecholamine Content

Treatment	Self-Stimulation (Percent Control)	Catecholamine Content (Percent Control)	
		NE	DA
α-Methyltyrosine (40 mg/kg)	48 ± 9*	54 ± 3*	41 ± 4*
U-14,624 (50 mg/kg)	94 ± 4	27 ± 6*	115 ± 18

Self-stimulation responding and catecholamine content were determined 4 hr after injection of α-methyltyrosine or U-14,624.
*$P < .001$ when compared with preinjection self-stimulation rate or control content of norepinephrine or dopamine.

Table 3

Effect of d-Amphetamine on Locus Coeruleus Responding in Reserpinized Rats Treated with α-Methyltyrosine or U-14,624

Treatment	Bar Press Response to Amphetamine Sulfate (1.0 mg/kg)
	Responses/75 min
Reserpine	2188 ± 714
Reserpine + α-Methyltyrosine (25 mg/kg)	6 ± 3*
Reserpine + U-14,624 (50 mg/kg)	2433 ± 544

Rats were assigned to groups so that they were matched for rates of self-stimulation prior to reserpine treatment (2.5 mg/kg, s.c.). Rats received α-methyltyrosine (25 mg/kg, i.p.) or U-14,624 (50 mg/kg) 1 hr before receiving 1 mg/kg of amphetamine.
*$P < .001$ when compared with reserpine group.

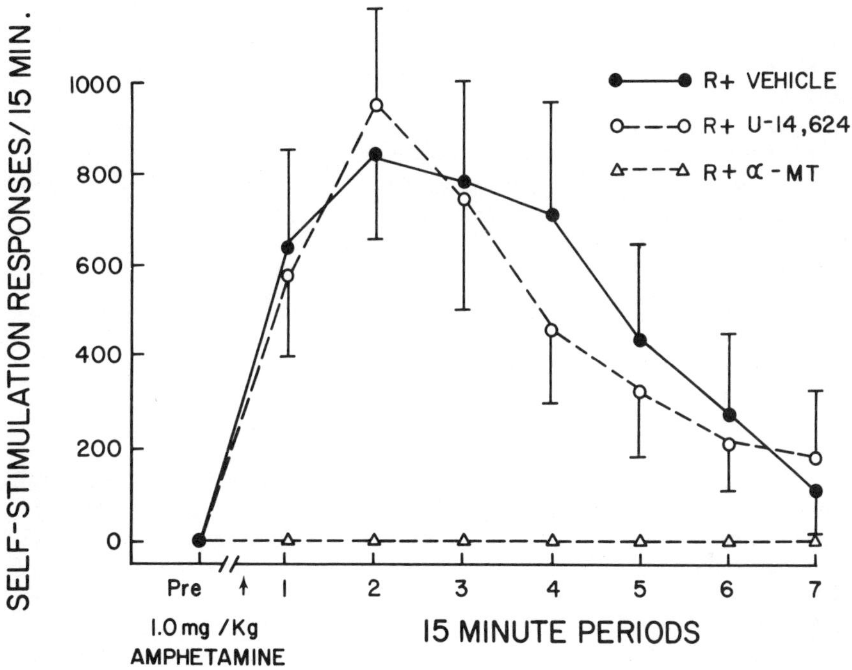

Fig. 5. Effects of d-amphetamine on lateral hypothalamic self-stimulation responding in reserpinized rats treated with either α-methyltyrosine or U-14,624. Rats received reserpine (R; 2.5 mg/kg) 24 hr before receiving α-methyltyrosine (α-MT; 25 mg/kg) or U-14,624 (50 mg/kg). One hr after these treatments animals received d-amphetamine sulfate (1 mg/kg).

point to a role for dopaminergic neurons in responding maintained by electrodes placed in this "noradrenergic" site. Curiously, evidence which would implicate norepinephrine has not, as yet, been obtained.

Summary

The studies described provide compelling evidence that dopaminergic neural systems have an important function in maintaining self-stimulation. From studies of animals with electrodes implanted in the lateral hypothalamus, the depressant effects of α-methyltyrosine were found to be significantly potentiated in rats in which brain dopamine was reduced - an observation not evident in control rats or in animals in which brain norepinephrine has been preferentially reduced. By administering a dopamine-β-hydroxylase inhibitor to animals with noradrenergic content reduced with 6-hydroxydopamine, we attempted to examine the possibility that destruction of brain noradrenergic fibers was not sufficient to produce a behavioral deficit. While an effect on self-stimulation was not observed, the possible involvement of dopamine accumulation and release from noradrenergic fibers in animals treated with a dopamine-β-hydroxylase inhibitor must not be ignored (Andén et al., 1973). However, any such interpretation will be confounded by the observation that norepinephrine infusion into brain will facilitate self-stimulation of the lateral hypothalamus whereas dopamine administration will not (Wise and Stein, 1969).

Earlier studies have used drugs that facilitate self-stimulation to imply the neurochemical basis of this phenomenon (Poschel and Ninteman, 1963; Stein, 1964; Crow, 1972). In the present work, the d-amphetamine-induced increase in self-stimulation from the lateral hypothalamus was reduced by treatments that interrupted the function of dopaminergic fibers but not by procedures that interfered with function of noradrenergic fibers. Thus, these data suggest that d-amphetamine facilitates self-stimulation responding by releasing brain dopamine and implicate further brain dopaminergic fibers in the maintenance of intracranial self-stimulation. Such findings would also be consistent with evidence which has implicated dopamine in locomotor stimulation produced by d-amphetamine (Breese et al., 1973; Hollister et al., 1974).

Perhaps the most surprising finding was that locus coeruleus self-stimulation was affected very much like that obtained from the lateral hypothalamus. Since the locus coeruleus is not known to contain any dopaminergic cell bodies or pathways (Dahlstrom and Fuxe, 1964; Ungerstedt, 1971), it is presently difficult to comprehend the anatomical basis of these results. One possible explanation would be that noradrenergic fibers are not involved in the maintenance of self-stimulation and that this anatomical pathway is coincident with another neural system which would, at least in the dorsal tegmentum, have to be something other than dopaminergic. The studies of Thalmann (1974) which indicate that self-stimulation of the dorsal tegmentum may be maintained by large myelinated fibers would be in accord with this latter suggestion. This might explain the fact that drugs which influence other transmitter systems can also affect self-stimulation (Domino and Olds, 1968; Wise et al., 1973). An additional possibility is that self-stimulation is disrupted by reduction of dopamine in the basal ganglia, resulting in a decreased ability to perform the bar press task for brain stimulation. Perhaps this interpretation would apply as well to other studies in which destruction of brain dopaminergic pathways has been found to disrupt behavior (Ungerstedt and Ljüngberg, 1973; Breese, 1973; Breese et al., 1975; Cooper and Breese, 1974). The answer to these questions will only be found in future research.

Acknowledgements

This work was supported by U.S.P.H.S. grants MH-16522, HD-03110, and MH-15631. G.R.B. is supported by a Career Development Award (MH-00013). The authors acknowledge the excellent assistance of Joseph Farmer, Marcine Kindead, Susan Hollister and Edna Edwards.

References

Andén, N. E., Atack, C.V. and Svensson, T.H.: Release of dopamine from central noradrenaline and dopamine nerves induced by a dopamine-β-hydroxylase inhibitor. J. Neural Transmission 34: 93-100, 1973.

Arbuthnott, G.W., Crow, T.J., Fuxe, K., Olson, L. and Ungerstedt, U.: Depletion of catecholamines induced by electrical stimulation of central monoamine pathways. Brain Res. 24: 471-483, 1970.

Black, W.C. and Cooper, B.R.: Reduction of electrically rewarded behavior by interference with monoamine synthesis. Psychol. Behav. 5: 1405-1409, 1970.

Breese, G.R.: Chemical and immunochemical lesions by specific neurotoxic substances and antisera. In Handbook of Psychopharmacology, ed. by L.L. Iversen, S.D. Iversen and S.H. Snyder, pp. 137-174, Plenum Press, New York, 1975.

Breese, G.R., Cooper, B.R. and Hollister, A.S.: Relationship of biogenic amines to behavior. J. Psychiat. Res. 11: 125-133, 1974.

Breese, G.R., Cooper, B.R. and Smith, R.D.: Biochemical and behavioral alterations following 6-hydroxydopamine administration into brain. In Frontiers in Catecholamine Research, ed. by E. Usdin and S. Snyder, pp. 701-706, Pergamon Press, New York, 1973.

Breese, G.R., Howard, J. and Leahy, P.: Effect of 6-hydroxydopamine on electrical self-stimulation of brain. Brit. J. Pharmacol. 43: 255-257, 1971.

Breese, G.R. and Traylor, T.D.: Effect of 6-hydroxydopamine on brain norepinephrine and dopamine: evidence for selective degeneration of catecholamine neurons. J. Pharmacol. Exp. Ther. 174: 413-420, 1970.

Breese, G.R. and Traylor, T.D.: Depletion of brain noradrenaline and dopamine by 6-hydroxydopamine. Brit. J. Pharmacol. 42: 88-99, 1971.

Cooper, B.R., Breese, G.R., Grant, L.D. and Howard, J.L.: Effects of 6-hydroxydopamine treatments on active avoidance responding: evidence for involvement of brain dopamine. J. Pharmacol. Exp. Therap. 185: 358-370, 1973.

Cooper, B.R., Breese, G.R., Howard, J.L. and Grant, L.D.: Enhanced behavioral depressant effects of reserpine and α-methyltyrosine after 6-hydroxydopamine treatment. Psychopharmacologia 27: 99-110, 1972.

Cooper, B.R., Cott, J.M. and Breese, G.R.: Effects of catecholamine-depleting drugs and amphetamine on self-stimulation of brain following various 6-hydroxydopamine treatments. Psychopharmacologia 37: 235-248, 1974.

Crow, T.J.: Mode of enhancement of self-stimulation in rats by methamphetamine. Nature (Lond.) 224: 709-710, 1969.

Crow, T.J.: Enhancement by cocaine of intra-cranial self-stimulation in the rat. Life Sciences 9: 375-381, 1970.

Crow, T.J.: Catecholamine-containing neurons and electrical self-stimulation. I. A review of some data. Psychol. Med. 2: 414-421, 1972.

Crow, T.J., Spear, P.J., Arbuthnott, G.: Intracranial self-stimulation with electrodes in the region of the locus coeruleus. Brain Res. 36: 275-287, 1972.

Dahlstrom, A. and Fuxe, K.: Evidence for the existence of monoamine neurons in the central nervous system. I. Demonstration of monoamines in the cell bodies of brain stem neurons. Acta Physiol. Scand. 62: Suppl. 232, 1-55, 1964.

Deutsch, J.A. and Howarth, C.I.: Some tests of a theory of intracranial self-stimulation. Psychol. Rev. 70: 444-460, 1963.

Domino, E.F. and Olds, M.E.: Cholinergic inhibition of self-stimulation behavior. J. Pharmacol. Exp. Ther. 164: 202-211, 1968.

Fuxe, K.: Evidence for the existence of monoamine neurons in the central nervous system. IV. Distribution of monoamine nerve terminals in the central nervous system. Acta Physiol. Scand. 64: Suppl. 247, 39-85, 1965.

Fuxe, K. and Jonsson, G.: Further mapping of central 5-HT neurons: Studies with the neurotoxic dihydroxytryptamines. Advances in Biochemical Pharmacology. 10: 1-12, 1974.

Gibson, S., McGeer, E.G. and McGeer, P.L.: Effect of selective inhibitors of tyrosine and tryptophan hydroxylases on self-stimulation in the rat. Exp. Neurol. 27: 283-290, 1970.

Hanson, L.C.F.: Evidence that the central action of amphetamine is mediated via catecholamines. Psychopharmacologia 9: 78-80, 1966.

Hollister, A.S., Breese, G.R. and Cooper, B.R.: Comparison of tyrosine hydroxylase and dopamine-β-hydroxylase inhibition with the effects of various 6-hydroxydopamine treatments on amphetamine-induced motor activity. Psychopharmacologia 36: 1-16, 1974.

Liebman, J.M. and Butcher, L.L.: Effects on self-stimulation behavior of drugs influencing dopaminergic neurotransmission mechanisms. Nauyn-Schmiedeberg's Arch. Pharmacol. 277: 306-318, 1973.

Lippa, A.S., Antelman, S.M., Fischer, A.E. and Canfield, D.R.: Neurochemical mediation of reward: A significant role for dopamine? Pharmacol. Biochem. Behav. 1: 23-28, 1973.

Miller, N.E.: Some reflections on the law of effect produce a new alternative to drive reduction. In Nebraska Symposium on Motivation, ed. by M.R. Jones, pp. 65-112, University of Nebraska Press, Lincoln, 1963.

Olds, J.: Self-stimulation experiments and differentiated reward systems. In The Reticular Formation of the Brain, ed. by H.H. Jasper, L.D. Proctor, R.S. Knighton, W.C. Noshay and R.T. Costello, pp. 671-687, Little Brown, Boston, 1958.

Olds, J.: Hypothalamic substrates of reward. Physiol. Rev. 42: 554-604, 1962.

Olds, J. and Milner, P.: Positive reinforcement produced by electrical stimulation of septal area and other regions of rat brain. J. Comp. Physiol. Psych. 47: 419-427, 1954.

Olds, J. and Travis, R.P.: Effects of chlorpromazine, meprobamate, pentobarbital and morphine on self-stimulation. J. Pharmacol. Exp. Ther. 128: 397-404, 1960.

Phillips, A.G. and Fibiger, H.: Dopaminergic and noradrenergic substrates of positive reinforcement: Differential effects of d- and l-amphetamine. Science 179: 575-577, 1973.

Poschel, B.P.H.: Mapping of rat brain for self-stimulation under monoamine oxidase blockade. Physiol. Behav. 4: 325-331, 1969.

Poschel, B.P.H. and Ninteman, F.W.: Norepinephrine: A possible excitatory neurohormone of the reward system. Life Sciences 1: 782-788, 1963.

Poschel, B.P.H. and Ninteman, F.W.: Excitatory (antidepressant) effects of monoamine oxidase inhibitors on the reward system of the brain. Life Sciences 3: 903-910, 1964.

Poschel, B.P.H. and Ninteman, F.W.: Hypothalamic self-stimulation: Its suppression by blockade of norepinephrine biosynthesis and reinstatement by methamphetamine. Life Sciences 5: 11-16, 1966.

Randrup, A. and Scheel-Krüger, J.: Diethyldithiocarbamate and amphetamine stereotype behavior. J. Pharm. Pharmacol. 18: 752, 1966.

Ritter, S. and Stein, L.: Self-stimulation of noradrenergic cell group (A6) in locus coeruleus of rats. J. Comp. Physiol. Psychol. 85: 443-452, 1973.

Roll, S.K.: Intracranial self-stimulation and wakefulness: Effect of manipulating ambient brain catecholamines. Science 168: 1370-1372, 1970.

Stein, L.: Effects and interactions of imipramine, chlorpromazine, reserpine, and amphetamine on self-stimulation: Possible neurophysiological basis of depression. Rec. Adv. Biol. Psychiat. 4: 288-309, 1962.

Stein, L.: Self-stimulation of the brain and the central stimulant action of amphetamine. Federation Proc. 23: 836-850, 1964.

Stein, L.: Psychopharmacological substrates of mental depression. In International Symposium on Antidepressant Drugs, ed. by M. Dukes, pp. 130-140, Excerpta Medica Foundation, Amsterdam, 1967.

Stein, L.: Chemistry of reward and punishment. In Psychopharmacology: A Review of Progress (1957-1967), ed. by D. Efron, pp. 105-123, U.S. Government Printing Office, Washington, D.C., 1968.

Stein, L. and Wise, C.D.: Release of norepinephrine from hypothalamus and amygdala by rewarding medial forebrain bundle stimulation and amphetamine. J. Comp. Physiol. Psych. 67: 189-198, 1969.

Stein, L. and Wise, C.D.: Possible etiology of schizophrenia: Progressive damage to the noradrenergic reward system by 6-hydroxydopamine. Science 171: 1032-1036, 1971.

Stein, L. and Wise, D.: Amphetamine and noradrenergic reward pathways. In Frontiers in Catecholamine Research, ed. by E. Usdin and S. Snyder, pp. 963-968, Pergamon Press, New York, 1973.

Taylor, K. and Snyder, S.: Amphetamine: Differentiation by d and l isomers of behavior involving brain norepinephrine or dopamine. Science 168: 1487, 1970.

Taylor, K.M. and Snyder, S.H.: Differential effects of d- and l-amphetamine on behavior and on catecholamine disposition in dopamine and norepinephrine containing neurons of rat brain. Brain Res. 28: 295-309, 1971.

Thalmann, R.H.: Self-stimulation of the dorsal midbrain as a function of the interval between conditioning and testing pulses. Abstracts for the Society for Neuroscience, p. 449, 1974.

Ungerstedt, U.: Stereotaxic mapping of the monoamine pathways in the rat brain. Acta Physiol. Scand. 367: 1-48, 1971.

Ungerstedt, U. and Ljüngberg, T.: Behavioral-anatomical correlates of brain catecholamines. In Frontiers in Catecholamine Research, Third International Catecholamine Symposium, ed. by E. Usdin and S. Snyder, pp. 689-693, Pergamon Press, London, 1973.

Uretsky, N.J. and Iversen, L.L.: Effects of 6-hydroxydopamine on catecholamine neurons in the rat brain. J. Neurochem. 17: 269-278, 1970.

Valenstein, E.S.: The anatomical locus of reinforcement. In Progress in Physiological Psychology, ed. by E. Stellar and J.M. Sprague, pp. 149-190, Academic Press, New York, 1966.

Wauquier, A. and Niemegeers, C.J.E.: Intracranial self-stimulation in rats as a function of various stimulus parameters. II. Influence of haloperidol, pimozide, and pipamperone on medial forebrain bundle stimulation with monopolar electrodes. Psychopharmacologia 27: 191-202, 1972.

Weissman, A., Koe, B.K. and Tenen, S.S.: Antiamphetamine effects following inhibition of tyrosine hydroxylase. J. Pharmacol. Exp. Ther. 151: 339-352, 1966.

Wise, C.D., Berger, B.D. and Stein, L.: Evidence of α-noradrenergic reward receptors and serotonergic punishment receptors in rat brain. Biol. Psych. 6: 3-21, 1973.

Wise, C.D. and Stein, L.: Facilitation of brain self-stimulation by central administration of norepinephrine. Science 163: 299-301, 1969.

Neurotransmitter Balances Regulating Behavior, edited and published by E.F. Domino and J.M. Davis, Ann Arbor, © 1975

ROLE OF NOREPINEPHRINE, DOPAMINE AND SEROTONIN IN REWARD MECHANISMS

B.P.H. Poschel and F.W. Ninteman
Parke, Davis and Company
Research and Development Division
Ann Arbor, Michigan

Any attempt to explain the role which monoamines play in intracranial reward must deal with two main questions. One is strictly empirical. What influences do the monoamines exert on self-stimulation behavior - excitatory, inhibitory or none? The second question is mainly theoretical. Are the monoamine-containing neurons of the forebrain actual reinforcement neurons, or are they merely modulators of reinforcement thresholds?

Since 1970 our thinking on these questions has been the following: (a) Norepinephrine is excitatory to self-stimulation (Poschel and Ninteman, 1963; Stein, 1968). (b) Serotonin is inhibitory to self-stimulation (Poschel, 1970; Poschel and Ninteman, 1971). (c) The influence of norepinephrine and serotonin on self-stimulation is reciprocal (Poschel, 1970; Poschel and Ninteman, 1971). (d) Dopamine is essential to motor function and in this way enters into self-stimulation behavior, but not into the underlying reward process *per se*. This notion is the most tentative of the present set, not being based solidly on experimental data, but mainly on circumstantial evidence (*cf*. Poschel and Ninteman, 1966) such as the fact that most of the brain's dopamine is concentrated in the corpus striatum. The best experimental evidence favoring the notion was provided by Wise and Stein (1969) who found that dopamine, in contrast to intraventricularly injected norepinephrine, did not reinstate disulfiram-suppressed self-stimulation. (e) The monoamine neurons of the forebrain are not actual reinforcement neurons, but serve only to modulate drive and reinforcement thresholds (Poschel, 1969). According to this view, other neurons or processes, as yet unidentified, mediate the actual reinforcing effects.

In recent work we have sought new ways to test these notions. The role of serotonin was tested further by means of 5,6-dihydroxytryptamine, a selective destroyer of serotonin-containing neurons. To be consistent with our views, 5,6-dihydroxytryptamine would have to produce an excitatory effect on self-stimulation, much like the excitatory effect we reported to occur after para-chlorophenylalanine (Poschel, 1970; Poschel and Ninteman, 1971). In other experiments, we studied the influence of the monoamine precursor substances L-DOPA and L-5HTP in rats pretreated with an extracerebral decarboxylase inhibitor. Moreover, by adding the use of a dopamine-beta-hydroxylase inhibitor in these experiments, we have been able to test rather directly the relative importance of dopamine versus norepinephrine in the self-stimulation phenomenon. Our purpose in this report is to summarize these new experiments. First let us deal with the 5,6-dihydroxytryptamine studies.

Studies of 5,6-dihydroxytryptamine

5,6-Dihydroxytryptamine (5,6-DHT) lowers brain serotonin levels by apparently selectively destroying serotonin-containing terminals and, possibly, axons (Baumgarten et al., 1971; Costa et al., 1972). If serotonin is inhibitory to self-stimulation, this drug should act to increase rates of self-stimulation.

Method. Male albino Holtzman rats were implanted with a single self-stimulation electrode aimed at the medial forebrain bundle just anterior to the mammillary bodies. Each electrode was monopolar and made of 30-gauge platinum wire with the final 0.5 mm of the tip bared of insulation. The indifferent electrode pole was soldered to a stainless steel screw secured to the skull. Each rat was also implanted with a permanent cannula aimed at the lateral ventricle on the side opposite to the electrode. The cannulae were made from 21-gauge stainless steel hypodermic needles. At the completion of behavioral testing, the actual placement of all electrode and cannula tips was determined from enlarged photographs of frozen sections of the brains.

Starting about 2-3 weeks after surgery, the rats were trained to press a lever to stimulate their brains electrically. Each press of the lever delivered 60 Hz sine wave stimulation, 0.4 sec in duration. After the rats became expert in self-stimulation responding, the current was gradually lowered to medium levels to produce moderate but stable base line rates of response. The total training time of the animals took about 7 weeks.

In the critical tests, each daily self-stimulation session was at least 7 hr long. Intraventricular injections were administered 1 hour into a session, using 10 μl of Ringer-Locke solution as the carrier. Each rat's response to just Ringer-Locke solution was tested first. About 1 week later the response to 5,6-DHT (50 μg; creatinine sulfate dihydrate; dose calculated as free base) was tested, and the rats were also then run without further injections for the next 3 consecutive days.

Results and Discussion. Ten rats were tested in the above procedure. Seven of these rats developed a large excitatory effect, 6 of them 24 hr after, and one of them 72 hr after drug treatment. The 72 hr delay in the one rat appeared to be explained by the fact that its cannula had not entered the lateral ventricle, and thus the 5,6-DHT had been injected intracerebrally, rather than intraventricularly.

The effect of the 5,6-DHT treatment in these 7 rats is depicted in figure 1, which shows the mean number of self-stimulations the rats made in each 7 hr test session. The

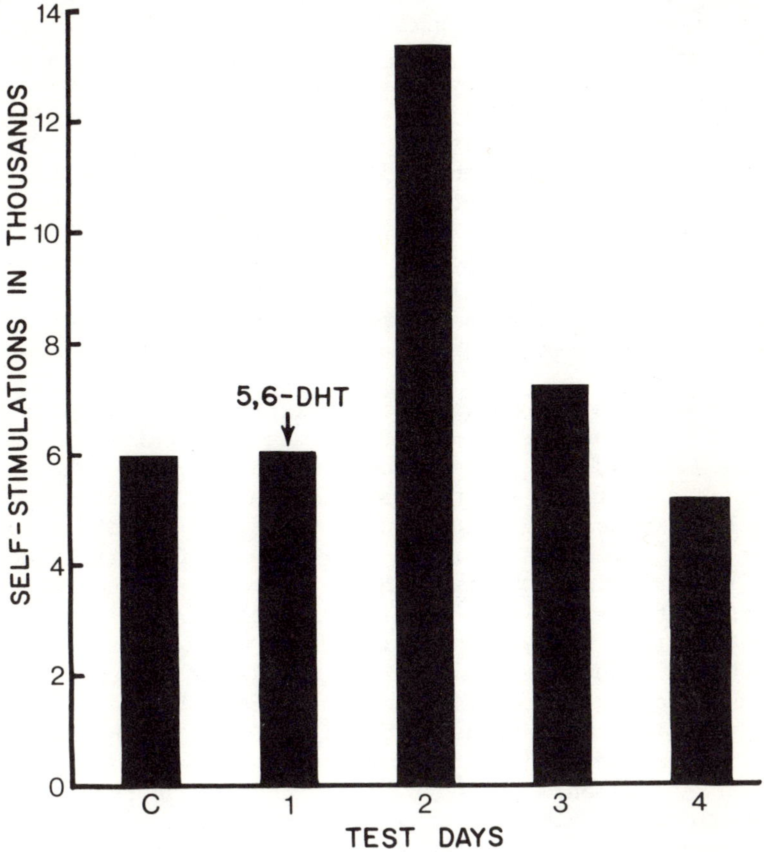

Fig. 1. Mean number of self-stimulations per day (7 hr sessions) before and after intraventricular 5,6-DHT (50 μg). Treatment given 1 hr into indicated session. On control (C) day, just Ringer-Locke solution was administered.

large effect seen on test day 2, 24 hr after 5,6-DHT treatment, was significant compared to the control day (*t*= 3.22, *df*=6, $P < .01$; one-tailed test). No statistically significant effects occurred on the other test days.

The relatively rapid fall off of the excitatory effect shown in figure 1 was somewhat surprising to us. However, the rate of disappearance of the behavioral effect was completely consistent with the changes in whole brain serotonin which occurred under our conditions. This was shown by chemical studies.

In these chemical studies, 4 groups of 10 rats were employed. The groups were matched very closely for mean body weight with the rats in the self-stimulation experiment. In short, all conditions between the original self-stimulation experiment and the present chemical study were matched as closely as possible. Two of the 4 groups of rats were injected stereotaxically in the lateral ventricle with 5,6-DHT (50 µg), and killed by decapitation 24 or 72 hr later. The third group was injected intraventricularly with Ringer-Locke solution alone, and killed 24 hr later. The fourth group was not treated at all prior to sacrifice. The whole brains were removed within 2 min after decapitation and frozen in crushed dry ice. The brains were stored at -70°C for 3-7 days before analysis for dopamine, norepinephrine, and serotonin, using the respective methods of Anton and Sayre (1964), Euler and Lishajko (1959), and Maickel *et al.* (1968).

The results are shown in table 1, expressed as mean µg/g of brain tissue ± S.E. Comparing the results in the first two rows shows that Ringer-Locke solution *per se* had no effect on any of the monoamines. The third row shows the levels of monoamines occurring 1 day after 5,6-DHT treatment, the time when we found the large excitatory effect on self-stimulation. Brain dopamine was not affected at all. Norepinephrine was reduced significantly, but only slightly in percentage terms. The main effect was on serotonin, which was reduced by 40%. Thus, the large increase in self-stimulation rate seen in figure 1 was associated with a fairly selective decline in brain serotonin. The last row of table 1 shows the effects occurring 3 days after the 5,6-DHT treatment. Here serotonin levels had recovered much closer to normal, being only 16.6% less than the control level. Figure 1 showed at this time self-stimulation rate had returned essentially to normal. Thus, we have very good agreement between the self-stimulation effects and the chemical effects. 5,6-DHT caused a substantial decline in brain serotonin levels and this was associated with a large increase in rates of self-stimulation. Later,

Table 1

Effect of 5,6-DHT on Rat Whole Brain Monoamines

Intraventricular Treatment	μg/g brain tissue		
	5-HT	NE	DA
None	.534 $\pm$ .019	.541 $\pm$ .014	.774 $\pm$ .023
Ringer-Locke	.548 $\pm$ .016	.561 $\pm$ .015	.733 $\pm$ .029
50 μg 5,6-DHT 24 hr prior	.328 $\pm$ .020[a]	.487 $\pm$ .013[b]	.771 $\pm$ .028
50 μg 5,6-DHT 72 hr prior	.457 $\pm$ .016[a]	.491 $\pm$ .026[b]	.868 $\pm$ .041[b]

[a]P < .001; *t* tests against Ringer-Locke treated groups.
[b]P < .05; *t* tests against Ringer-Locke treated groups.

when serotonin levels had risen close to normal, the excitatory effect on self-stimulation was lost.

The obvious conclusion is that serotonin is an inhibitory substance to self-stimulation. Most investigators, we think, judging from the research literature, would be content with this statement, offering no qualifications for the statement. Unfortunately, the self-stimulation phenomenon is not that simple, a qualification is needed, one pertaining to electrode placement. We have seen the importance of electrode placement repeatedly in pharmacological studies of the self-stimulation phenomenon, and the present study with 5,6-DHT is another case in point.

Thus, in the present study 10 rats in all were employed. Seven showed an excitatory effect, while 3 did not. What factor determined whether or not the excitatory effect showed up? We think the critical factor was electrode placement. Figure 2 documents this belief.

Figure 2 shows the electrode placement in each of the 10 rats in the study. The electrode tips are drawn to scale to show exactly the region in the brain stimulated. In addition, the rats are numbered in a rank-order manner, indicating the magnitude of the percent increase in self-stimulation rate obtained after 5,6-DHT. Thus, rat number 1 had the largest excitatory effect, and rat number 7 had the smallest excitatory effect. Rats 8, 9, and 10 were the 3 rats with no excitatory effect at all. Each of these 3 rats was a good self-stimulator, even though the electrode tip missed the medial forebrain bundle where serotonin-containing axons are concentrated as they ascend to higher regions of the brain. Thus, it appears that these serotonin-containing neurons are not essential to self-stimulation, but they are essential to the excitatory effect normally seen after 5,6-DHT. Significantly, as we might expect, the first 7 rats had their electrode tips right in those regions rich in the serotonin-containing neurons, that is, in the medial forebrain bundle or the ventral tegmental area of Tsai. The conclusion we must draw is that the self-stimulation phenomenon is not pharmacologically homogeneous. But this is not really surprising when we consider the fact that self-stimulation is obtained from such large and diverse areas of the brain.

Studies of L-DOPA and L-5HTP

Method. The behavioral method in these experiments was essentially the same as in the studies just described. However, in the present experiments the rats did not have intraventricular cannulae, and all drugs were administered

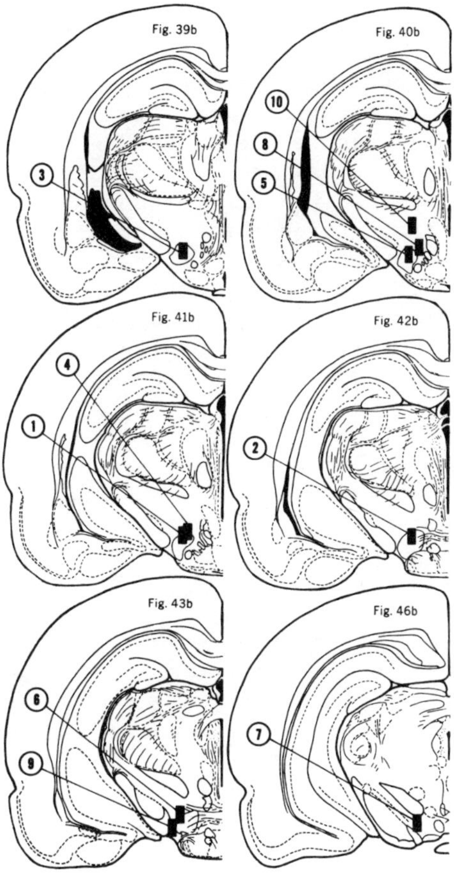

Fig. 2. Drawings of rat brain based on Konig and Klippel (1963) showing location of electrode tips of rats in 5,6-DHT study. Electrode tips drawn to scale. Numbers identifying rats also serve as rank-order measure of percent increase in self-stimulation obtained 24-hr posttreatment (test day 2). In the case of rat No. 3 an exception was made because the injection went intracerebrally, and the peak action obtained 72 hr posttreatment was used for calculating this percent increase.

intraperitoneally. Isotonic saline or aqueous methocel were used as the drug vehicles.

The drugs employed and the dosing schedule were as follows. To block extracerebral decarboxylase we used 40 mg/kg of L-α-methyldopa hydrazine, also known as MK-486 (Bartholini and Pletscher, 1969; Messiha et al., 1972). Then, 90 min later, we administered the monoamine precursor substances L-DOPA (dihydroxyphenylalanine) or L-5HTP (5-hydroxytryptophane). Our dose of L-DOPA was usually 75 mg/kg, and our dose of L-5HTP was usually 84 mg/kg. These doses of L-DOPA and L-5HTP represent equal molar amounts; thus, the effects of the 2 substances can be directly compared. Finally, when we wished L-DOPA to produce a selective rise in brain dopamine, with little or no change in brain norepinephrine, we used the dopamine-β-hydroxylase inhibitor, diethyldithiocarbamic acid sodium (DEDTC) (Lippmann and Lloyd, 1969). Our dose of DEDTC was always 200 mg/kg, and it was usually administered 30 min prior to L-DOPA. The exact order and timing of these treatments will be made clear by figure 3 which shows a representative result obtained with this procedure.

Results and Discussion. All the self-stimulation records shown in figure 3 are from the same rat. Each record is 6 hr long, and each reset of the pen occurred after 550 self-stimulations. Record A shows the performance of the rat under the vehicle-control condition. Obviously the vehicles had no effect on self-stimulation. Record B shows the critical test of L-DOPA. The extracerebral decarboxylase inhibitor, MK-486, was administered 1 hr into the session. One hr later we gave a control injection of saline, and then 30 min after that, the injection of L-DOPA. There was no immediate effect of the DOPA but starting about 40 min later, a large excitatory effect developed which lasted for well over an hour and a half. The delay in the development of the effect undoubtedly represents the time required for conversion of L-DOPA to the catecholamines. Record C represents our attempt to determine which catecholamine is responsible for the excitatory effect seen in record B. Here we again gave our decarboxylase inhibitor, but then, at the 2 hr point, we gave the dopamine-β-hydroxylase inhibitor, DEDTC. Then, 30 min later we again gave L-DOPA. Under these conditions no excitatory effect developed. Therefore, the large excitatory effect seen in record B was, almost certainly, mainly dependent on norepinephrine, not on dopamine.

We know what was happening to monoamine levels in the brain under these conditions because the necessary chemical studies were run. These results will be shown a bit

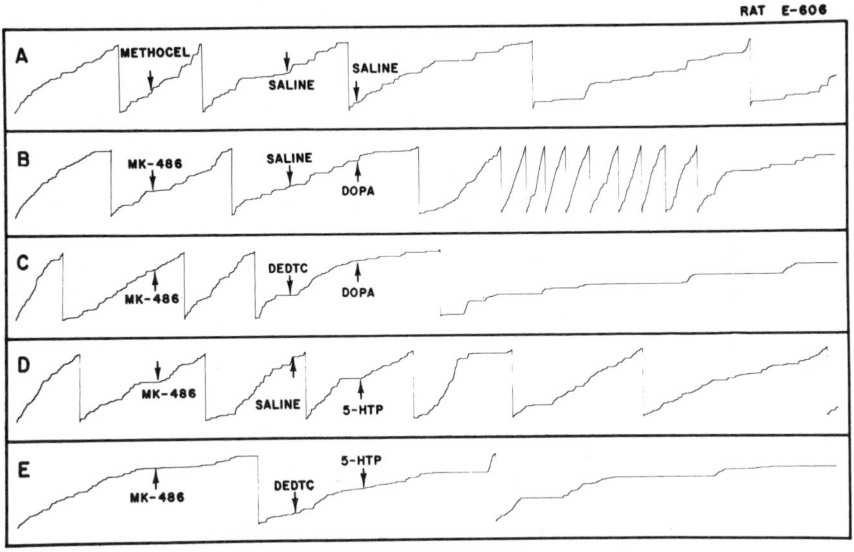

Fig. 3. Results of L-DOPA and L-5HTP experiments in rat E-606. Each record is 6 hr long and resets of recorder pen occurred after every 550 self-stimulations.

later. Suffice it now to say that under condition B, whole brain dopamine increased three and one-half times above normal, while norepinephrine increased two times above normal. However, under condition C, while whole brain dopamine still increased more than 3 times above normal, norepinephrine was virtually unaffected. Therefore, a selective large increase in whole brain dopamine levels does not suffice to produce the excitatory effect seen in record B, at least not in this rat. Norepinephrine, therefore, appears to be the critical amine.

Going on with the results in figure 3, record D shows that L-5HTP did not produce an excitatory effect on self-stimulation when the rat was pretreated with the extracerebral decarboxylase inhibitor. However, a depressant effect was not produced either, when we might have expected one if serotonin is inhibitory to self-stimulation. More will be said on this later when we consider where this rat's electrode was placed. Finally, record E shows that adding the dopamine-β-hydroxylase inhibitor to this experiment did not substantially change the result, as was expected. The only difference was that self-stimulation under condition E was somewhat depressed below the level seen under condition D. This result, of course, is understandable since the dopamine-β-hydroxylase inhibitor must have acted to reduce the level of newly synthesized norepinephrine.

Figure 4 (left) shows the electrode placement of the rat whose results we have just examined. The electrode was not in the medial forebrain bundle, which is very interesting. Rather the tip was above and to the right of the bundle, and just lateral to the mammillary-thalamic tract. This is an excellent locus for self-stimulation, as shown by the current level the rat worked for in these tests - 17.5 μA.

We can get some ideas as to why this is such a good self-stimulation point from the right-hand diagram shown in figure 4. This diagram was taken from Ungerstedt's (1971) mapping study of the monoamine pathways in the rat brain. This diagram represents a level in the brain which matches very closely our histological section. Now in Ungerstedt's diagram the fine dots represent the cross sections of serotonin-containing axons. These axons occupy primarily the ventral portion of the medial forebrain bundle. The heavy dots represent the cross sections of norepinephrine-containing neurons. These axons occupy primarily the dorsal portion of the bundle. The heavy striations represent norepinephrine-containing neurons seen longitudinally, that is, in their lengthwise dimension. Here is where our electrode tip was, right in the midst of the longitudinally-running norepinephrine axons. The histological data, therefore, support our pharmacological data; both sets of data indicate that norepinephrine is the excitatory monoamine for self-stimulation.

Incidentally, the norepinephrine axons we have been discussing represent what Ungerstedt (1971) calls the "dorsal norepinephrine bundle", which originates in the locus coeruleus. At the brain level shown in figure 4, this dorsal bundle is turning abruptly ventro-laterally to join the medial forebrain bundle. Then these axons travel up the medial forebrain bundle to innervate all areas of the cerebral cortex and the hippocampus.

There is one last important point to discuss regarding this electrode locus. We think it explains why 5-HTP failed to produce a depressant effect when tested in this animal. In short, the rat's electrode was so placed that it did not stimulate any serotonin-containing axons. Therefore, 5-HTP had no chance to influence this rat's self-stimulation behavior.

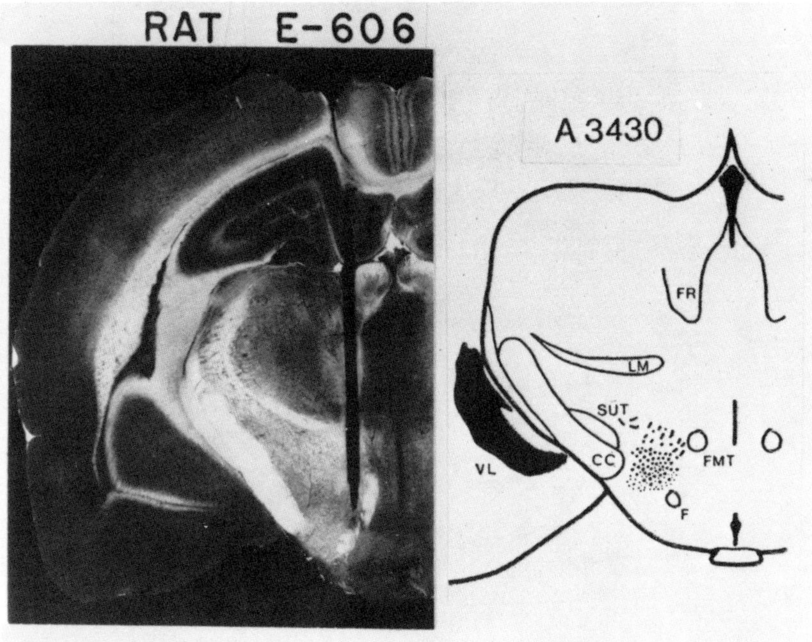

Fig. 4. Left: Histology of rat E-606 showing location of electrode tip. Right: Drawing of rat hypothalamic regions based on Ungerstedt (1971) showing fibers of dorsal norepinephrine bundle passing longitudinally through the region where rat E-606 had its electrode tip located.

The next question to ask is what would happen in this experiment if our electrode were placed so as also to activate serotonin axons. Such a locus, of course, is found in the medial forebrain bundle. The example shown in figure 5 is a case in point. This rat had its electrode right in the middle of the medial forebrain bundle, at a level where it had to influence norepinephrine axons of both the dorsal and ventral bundles, and also serotonin axons. There is also the possibility that it caught the edge of the dopamine pathway shown in Ungerstedt's (1971) diagram.

The results obtained with this rat are shown in figure 6. The drug conditions shown here are exactly the same as in

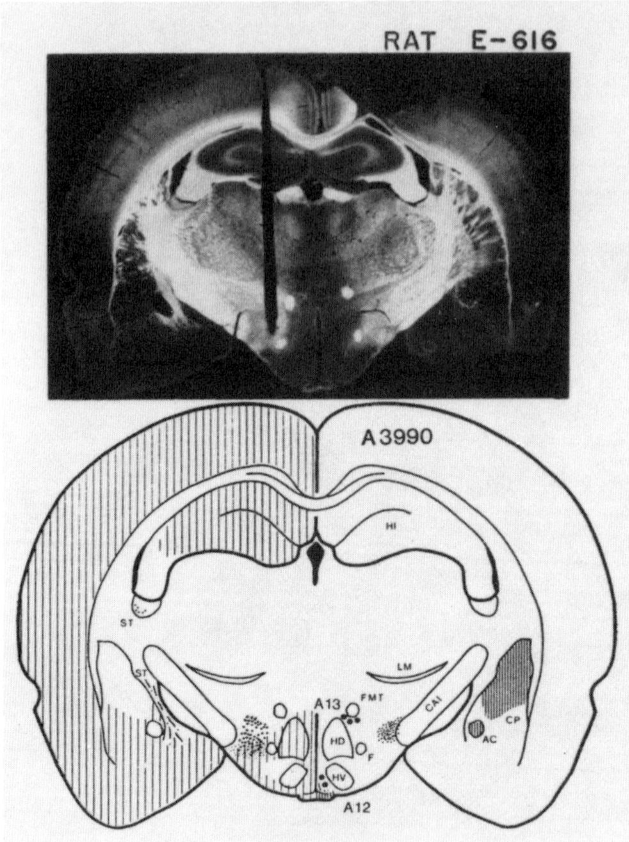

Fig. 5. Top: Histology of rat E-616 showing location of electrode tip. Bottom: Drawing of rat brain based on Ungerstedt (1971) showing norepinephrine and serotonin fibers passing transversely through the medial forebrain bundle where rat E-616 had its electrode tip located.

our previous example; this case differs from the earlier one only in terms of electrode placement. First, it should be noticed in record B that DOPA again produced a large excitatory effect, although not quite as large as in our earlier example. But an important aspect of these results is shown in record D. Here 5-HTP produced a small but clear inhibitory effect. The inhibitory effect is much more apparent in record E as, of course, it should have been because of the presence of dopamine-β-hydroxylase inhibitor. The inhibitory effect occurs in this rat, we think, because with its electrode placement serotonin axons in the medial forebrain bundle were activated by the intracranial stimu-

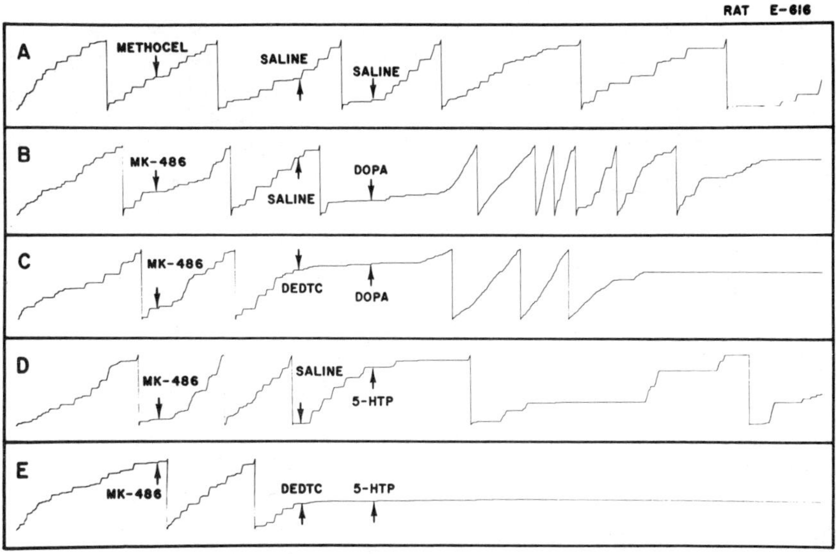

Fig. 6. Results of L-DOPA and L-5HTP experiments in rat E-616. Each record is 6 hr long and resets of recorder pen occurred after every 550 self-stimulations.

lation. This factor, we think, also explains why the excitatory effect seen in record B is not up to the level seen in our first example. In the present rat each press of the self-stimulation lever released both norepinephrine and serotonin at axon terminals, and the two amines would have produced reciprocally acting effects. In this reciprocal action, the norepinephrine effect obviously predominated, but not without cost to itself. This cost to the norepinephrine effect is shown in record B by L-DOPA producing only about half as large an excitatory effect as in our previous case, where a pure norepinephrine axon system was stimulated.

Finally, we should look at record C, where the dopamine-β-hydroxylase inhibitor was given prior to L-DOPA. Some excitatory effect did occur, although less than half that seen in record B. This again points up the importance of norepinephrine in self-stimulation. On the other hand, the fact that some excitation did occur could be important because it could represent a dopamine effect. You will recall that this rat's electrode tip was just on the edge of a dopamine axon system. In our first example, involving the rat with an electrode in a pure norepinephrine system, no effect at all was obtained under these conditions. So we don't think the effect seen here is just chance. For example, it could have arisen from dopaminergic stimulation of the motor processes involved in lever-pressing. We have not carried this work far enough to settle this particular issue. In any event, norepinephrine appears much more important than dopamine to the reward process per se, judging from our findings to date.

Finally, let us show you what happens to whole brain monoamine levels under the conditions of these experiments. This is shown in table 2. The results again are expressed as mean μg/g of brain tissue. The first row shows the vehicle control condition. The second row shows the effect of L-DOPA with extracerebral decarboxylase blocked. Dopamine levels went up 3 1/2 times. Norepinephrine levels doubled. Serotonin levels fell by 59%. The third row shows what happened when the additional condition of blockade of dopamine-β-hydroxylase was added to the experiment. Dopamine levels still went up very substantially--more than 3 times. Serotonin levels still fell a rather large amount --35%. But, significantly, norepinephrine levels remained almost unchanged. Thus, the dopamine-β-hydroxylase inhibitor did exactly what it was supposed to do--prevent a rise in brain norepinephrine levels after L-DOPA administration, without much affecting what happened to dopamine and serotonin levels. In short, the only monoamine which was differentially affected by the presence of the dopamine-β-hydroxylase inhibitor was norepinephrine. Thus, norepinephrine seemingly had to be mainly responsible for the excitatory effect observed in these experiments after L-DOPA administration.

Conclusions

Let us summarize the new findings that are reported in this paper.

1. The drug, 5,6-dihydroxytryptamine, when administered intraventricularly, produces an excitatory effect upon many self-stimulation points in the brain. This excitatory effect correlates biochemically with a reduction in whole brain serotonin.

2. The excitatory effect of 5,6-dihydroxytryptamine does not always occur--the effect depends on electrode placement.

Table 2

Effect of Inhibition of Extracerebral Decarboxylase and Dopamine-β-Hydroxylase on L-DOPA Induced Changes in Rat Whole Brain Monoamines

	μg/g brain tissue		
Treatment (I.P.)	DA	NE	5-HT
Methocel, Saline, Methocel	.965 ± .037	.418 ± .011	.476 ± .008
MK-486 (40 mg/kg), Saline, L-DOPA (75 mg/kg)	3.466 ± .060[a]	.835 ± .046[a]	.194 ± .009[a]
MK-486 (40 mg/kg), DEDTC (200 mg/kg), L-DOPA (75 mg/kg)	2.983 ± .095[a]	.440 ± .041	.311 ± .022[a]

[a]P <.001; t tests against methocel-saline-methocel treated groups.

Apparently, the determining factor is that the self-stimulation point under study must contain serotonin axons. Not all self-stimulation points have such serotonin axons. In general, the self-stimulation effects produced by 5,6-dihydroxytryptamine are similar to those produced by parachlorophenylalanine.

3. The monoamine precursor substances, L-DOPA and L-5HTP, produce large effects on self-stimulation in rats pretreated with an extracerebral decarboxylase inhibitor. Again, the exact nature of the effect produced on self-stimulation by these substances depends on electrode placement or, in other words, on the type of monoamine neurons which lie in close proximity to the electrode tip. In general, however, it is accurate to say that DOPA produces excitatory effects and 5HTP, inhibitory effects.

4. The use of a dopamine-β-hydroxylase inhibitor, administered prior to L-DOPA in these experiments, greatly clarifies the relative importance of dopamine and norepinephrine in the excitatory effect. For the self-stimulation points we have studied thus far, norepinephrine has always appeared much more important than dopamine. However, a critical experiment yet remains to be done. That is, to try this experiment with self-stimulation electrodes implanted in a region of the brain heavy in dopamine neurons but very light in the norepinephrine neurons. In rat brain, the region dorsal and lateral to the interpeduncular nucleus would serve such an experiment well.

Acknowledgment. The authors wish to thank Dr. J.R. McLean and Mrs. D. Potoczak for running the biochemical assays reported in tables 1 and 2.

References

Anton, A.H. and Sayre, D.F.: The distribution of dopamine and DOPA in various animals and a method for their determination in diverse biological material. J. Pharmacol. Exp. Ther. 145: 326-336, 1964.

Bartholini, G. and Pletscher, A.: Effect of various decarboxylase inhibitors on the cerebral metabolism of dihydroxyphenylalanine. J. Pharm. Pharmac. 21: 323-324, 1969.

Baumgarten, H.G., Bjorklund, A., Lachenmayer, L., Nobin, A. and Stenevi, U.: Long-lasting selective depletion of brain serotonin by 5,6-dihydroxytryptamine. Acta physiol. scand. Suppl. 373, 1-15, 1971..

Costa, E., LeFevre, H., Meek, J., Revuelta, A., Spano, F., Strada, S. and Daly, J.: Serotonin and catecholamine concentrations in brain of rats injected intracerebrally with 5,6-dihydroxytryptamine. Brain Res. 44: 304-308, 1972.

Euler, U.S.v. and Lishajko, F.: The estimation of catecholamines in urine. Acta physiol. scand. 45: 122-132, 1959.

Konig, J.F.R. and Kippel, R.A.: The Rat Brain. Williams and Wilkins, Baltimore, 1963.

Lippmann, W. and Lloyd, K.: Dopamine-β-hydroxylase inhibition by dimethyldithiocarbamate and related compounds. Biochem. Pharmac. 18: 2507-2516, 1969.

Maickel, R.P., Cox, R.H., Saillant, J. and Miller, F.P.: A method for the determination of serotonin and norepinephrine in discrete areas of rat brain. Int. J. Neuropharmacol. 7: 275-281, 1968.

Messiha, F.S., Hsu, T.H. and Bianchine, J.R.: Effects of peripheral aromatic L-amino acids decarboxylase inhibitor on L-[2-^{14}C]-3,4-dihydroxyphenylalanine metabolism in man. Biochem. Pharmac. 21: 2144-2147, 1972.

Poschel, B.P.H.: Mapping of rat brain for self-stimulation under monoamine oxidase blockade. Physiol. Behav. 4: 325-331, 1969.

Poschel, B.P.H.: Do the forebrain noradrenergic and serotonergic systems act reciprocally on self-stimulation? Paper read at the Amer. Psychol. Assoc. Symposium: Current Problems in Understanding Intracranial Self-Stimulation. Miami Beach, Florida, September, 1970.

Poschel, B.P.H. and Ninteman, F.W.: Norepinephrine: A possible excitatory neurohormone of the reward system. Life Sci. 2: 782-788, 1963.

Poschel, B.P.H. and Ninteman, F.W.: Hypothalamic self-stimulation: Its suppression by blockade of norepinephrine biosynthesis and reinstatement by methamphetamine. Life Sci. 5: 11-16, 1966.

Poschel, B.P.H. and Ninteman, F.W.: Intracranial reward and the forebrain's serotonergic mechanism: Studies employing para-chlorophenylalanine and para-chloroamphetamine. Physiol. Behav. 7: 39-46, 1971.

Stein, L.: Chemistry of reward and punishment. In Psychopharmacology, A Review of Progress 1957-1967, ed. by D.H. Efron, J.O. Cole, J. Levine and J.R. Wittenborn, Public Health Service Publication No. 1836, pp. 105-135, U.S. Government Printing Office, Washington, D.C., 1968.

Ungerstedt, U.: Stereotaxic mapping of the monoamine pathways in the rat brain. Acta physiol. scand. Suppl. 367, 1-48, 1971.

Wise, C.D. and Stein, L.: Facilitation of brain self-stimulation by central administration of norepinephrine. Science 163: 299-301, 1969.

Neurotransmitter Balances Regulating Behavior,
edited and published by E.F. Domino and
J.M. Davis, Ann Arbor, © 1975

BALANCES AMONG CENTRAL NEUROTRANSMITTERS IN SELF-STIMULATION BEHAVIOR

S.N. Pradhan
Howard University
College of Medicine
Washington, D.C.

In the peripheral autonomic nervous system there exists a balance between the effects of its two opposing components, sympathetic (adrenergic) and parasympathetic (cholinergic) on the organ systems, with adrenergic preponderance on the blood vessels and cholinergic preponderance on heart, smooth muscles and exocrine glands. In the event of induced alteration of function of some of these systems, a homeostasis mechanism operates to restore the activity to the normal level (e.g., baroreceptor mechanism for blood pressure regulation).

Within the central nervous system (CNS) similar reciprocal balance between opposing actions in the functional systems may also be demonstrated. According to the concept of Hess (1954), as presented by Brodie et al. (1959), the central adrenergic (ergotropic) and cholinergic (trophotropic) systems regulate the reactions of the animals to environmental changes by operating in continuous opposition. However, such balance within the CNS becomes complicated by the presence of a number of putative neurotransmitters; in addition to norepinephrine (NE) and acetylcholine (ACh), as in peripheral nervous system, there are also other transmitters, such as dopamine (DA), 5-hydroxytryptamine (5-HT), histamine and γ-aminobutyric acid that participate in modulation of various functions including behavior. Actions and interactions of several such transmitters with possible balance between them have been discussed with respect to a number of behaviors (Pradhan and Dutta, 1971; Izquierdo, 1972; Barbeau, 1972).

The nigrostriatal system is one of the important sites where balance of actions of several transmitters, particularly DA and ACh, and possibly others, has been observed pathologically as in Parkinson's disease as well as demonstrated experimentally in normal animals with respect to manifestations such as tremor, stereotypy and catalepsy. Furthermore, DA has been implicated to play a central role in controlling the balance between the various neurotransmitters present in the striatum; this balance involves both sensorimotor integration of the motor mechanism as well as regulation of central autonomic (both ergotropic and trophotropic) functions (Barbeau, 1972). A similar interaction between cholinergic and adrenergic systems has been indicated in hypothalamic thermoregulatory center of rats (Lomax et al., 1969).

The concept of balance within the CNS can be further substantiated to some extent by interactions of the agents related to the central neurotransmitters and their antagonists. A few examples can be cited from a large number of relevant investigations. Thus, central cholinergic blockade by atropine and scopolamine was demonstrated to increase several central effects of amphetamine (including those on motor activity and shock avoidance). On the other hand, central cholinergic stimulation antagonized the effect of amphetamine on motor activity (Carlton, 1961; Carlton and Didamo, 1961; Mennear, 1965; Ray and Bivens, 1968). In other studies, Ho and his associates (Ho et al., 1971; Ho and Loh, 1972) observed an increase in choline acetylase (ChA) activity (as an indication of the level of cholinergic activity) in certain areas of the brain following chronic central administration of NE and DA. On the other hand, ACh has been shown to increase the spontaneous release of catecholamines in the perfused cat brains (Glowinski, 1970; Philippu, 1970). Furthermore, diisopropyl phosphofluoridate (DFP), an anticholinesterase, caused a decrease in the level of NE in the diencephalon-midbrain area of rabbits pretreated with L-DOPA and a MAO inhibitor. This effect of DFP could be antagonized by atropine (Glisson et al., 1972).

Self-stimulation is a positively reinforced (rewarded) behavior in which the subject electrically stimulates itself at the site of electrode implantation within the brain by pressing a bar. The positively reinforcing nature of the behavior is indicated by making the animal repeat the bar-pressing response that immediately precedes the stimulus. In the rat, such positively reinforcing sites have been demonstrated in various brain areas extending from the forebrain to the rostral pons, most prominent among them being the medial forebrain bundle in the posterior lateral hypothalamus (Olds, 1958, 1962).

Neurochemical, neurohistochemical and neuropharmacological approaches have demonstrated involvement of several putative central neurotransmitters in self-stimulation behavior. NE and possibly DA have been implicated to play a facilitatory role, while ACh and 5-HT exert inhibitory influences. A question then arises whether the individual transmitters that affect this behavior would do so by acting separately in insulated structural or functional compartments or by interacting with each other to varying extents and by establishing a balance between them. The objective of this presentation is to review the works of a number of investigators including ours to discuss the actions and interactions of NE, DA, ACh and 5-HT on self-stimulation in an attempt to determine the role of balance between their actions in modulation of this behavior.

II. Role of Various Neurotransmitter Mechanisms in Self-Stimulation

(i) Role of Noradrenergic Mechanism

A number of reviews (Olds, 1962; Stein, 1964, 1968; Pradhan and Dutta, 1971) on self-stimulation behavior have indicated that the drugs that influence central adrenergic mechanism have their most marked and selective effects on this reward system. Drugs and chemicals affecting catecholamine (CA) metabolism also affect self-stimulation responding, presumably altering the effective CA concentration at the receptor site. Such correlation has been the subject matter of a large number of investigations. To avoid a lengthy presentation, data from some of these experiments are summarized in Table 1.

It appears from the table that the drugs and chemicals that enhance, release or inhibit re-entry or oxidation and thereby increase concentration of NE at the receptor sites, also increase self-stimulation responding. Reversely, the agents that inhibit synthesis or deplete the stores of NE, block the noradrenergic receptor sites or degenerate the central CA-containing neurons and thereby decrease the effective concentration of NE at the receptor site also decrease self-stimulation responding. However, certain items in the table need some comments. The effects of dopamine-β-hydroxylase (DBH) inhibitors have been to some extent controversial. Wise and Stein (1969) demonstrated a reduction of self-stimulation responding following administration of certain DBH inhibitors (e.g., disulfiram, diethyl dithio-carbamate or DDC) and re-emphasized the role of NE in this behavior. This observation has been contradicted (Roll, 1970) and will be discussed later.

Table 1

Chemicals Affecting Catecholamine (CA) Metabolism and Self-Stimulation (SS) Responding

Chemicals	Effective CA conc. at receptor	SS respon-ding	Reference
Synthesis Inhibition	↓	↓	
α-Me-*p*-tyrosine			Poschel & Ninteman, 1966; Gibson *et al.*, 1970; Black & Cooper, 1970; Cooper *et al.*, 1971.
Disulfiram		*	Wise & Stein, 1969; Roll, 1970.
DDC			
Depletion of Stores	↓	↓	
Reserpine			Olds *et al.*, 1956; Olds, 1972.
Tetrabenazine			
Enhanced Release	↑	↑	
Amphetamine			Stein, 1964; Wise & Stein, 1969; Pradhan & Bowling, 1971.
α-Me-*m*-tyrosine			Crow, 1969; Poschel & Ninteman, 1963.
Inhibited Reentry	↑	↑	
Imipramine			Stein & Seifter, 1961.
Cocaine			Crow, 1970.
MAO Inhibitors	↑	↑	Poschel & Ninteman, 1964; Dresse, 1966a.
Adrenergic Blockade	↓	↓	
Phenoxybenzamine			
Propranolol			Bailey *et al.*, 1972.
Degeneration of Central CA-Containing Neurons	↓	↓	
6-OH-dopamine (l. vent.)			Breese et al., 1971; Stein & Wise, 1971.

*May be inhibited, but not abolished. ↑, increase; ↓, decrease.

Imipramine, an antidepressant drug that inhibits re-entry of NE into the storage site, depressed self-stimulation responding when the electric stimulus was set just above the threshold level. However, when the stimulus was set below threshold, it was not efficacious. Under this condition, amphetamine caused self-stimulation to occur and imipramine markedly facilitated amphetamine-induced responding (Stein and Seifter, 1961).

(ii) Role of Dopaminergic Mechanism

Although the previous discussion describes NE as the sole facilitatory neurotransmitter in self-stimulation, recently DA has also been ascribed to such a role in addition to or even sometimes in place of NE. Such a role of DA has been substantiated at least three different ways: a) by maintaining the self-stimulation responding after blockade of synthesis of NE from DA by using inhibitors of DA-β-hydroxylase, b) by establishing self-stimulation responding with electrodes at sites containing only DA cells, and c) by analysis of actions of drugs that affect DA metabolism and act on central DA receptors.

a) <u>DBH inhibitors as tools for exploration</u>. In contradiction to the observation of Wise and Stein (1969) described earlier, Roll (1970) reported that following treatment with disulfiram (100 mg/kg) the self-stimulating rats appeared sedated and slow in bar-pressing but would always resume bar-pressing at normal rate if handled and replaced on the bar. This led to the conclusion that decrease in responding might be due to the effect of the DBH inhibitor on wakefulness rather than on motivation for or reward from self-stimulation and NE may not be necessary for self-stimulation. Leibman and Butcher (1973) also observed a reduction in self-stimulation responding under normal current after 150 mg/kg of disulfiram, but the rates were reinstated to greater than control level by doubling the current. These authors feel that disulfiram-induced inhibition does not appear to be due to non-specific sedative effect or motor incapacity.

b) <u>Dopaminergic neuronal system</u>. Crow (1972a, 1973) demonstrated that, in addition to the NE-containing neuronal systems described earlier, self-stimulation behavior could be established with stimulating electrodes in a ventral area in the mesencephalon surrounding the interpeduncular nucleus and extending into the pars compacta of the substantia nigra and also a limited dorsal area located at a point just lateral to the central grey matter. This ventral mesencephalic area corresponds closely to areas A9 and A10 of Dahlström and Fuxe (1965), consisting of DA-containing cell bodies sending out axons that travel rostrally via medial forebrain bundle to be distributed to the corpus striatum and other areas.

c) Drugs affecting DA receptors. Detailed scrutinization of effects of the drugs listed in Table 1 shows that dopaminergic neurotransmission is also affected by d-amphetamine (Munkvad et al., 1968), cocaine (Fog, 1969), MAO inhibitors (Carlsson, 1964), reserpine (Carlsson, 1964), α-methyl p-tyrosine (Rech et al., 1966), and chlorpromazine (Janssen et al., 1968; Andén et al., 1970). Moreover, the facilitatory effects on self-stimulation can be elicited by both d- and l-isomers of amphetamine with electrodes not only at the lateral hypothalamus which contains both noradrenergic and dopaminergic fibers but also at the substantia nigra that solely contains dopaminergic cell bodies. In this respect, while the d-isomer was 7-10 times more effective than the l-isomer at the hypothalamic site, the two isomers were equipotent at the substantia nigra (Phillips and Fibiger, 1973). In another study (Canfield et al., 1973), d-amphetamine alone or in combination with FLA-63, a DBH inhibitor (25 mg/kg, i.p.) caused the same increase in self-stimulation responding on a VI-15 sec schedule, while FLA-63 itself did not show any effect.

Self-stimulation behavior has been shown to be modified by drugs affecting DA receptors. Thus, phenothiazines and butyrophenones, neuroleptics which block DA receptors, inhibit self-stimulation (Dresse, 1966a,b; Stark et al., 1969; Wauquier and Neimegeers, 1972). Pimozide, another neuroleptic which at low dose (0.5 mg/kg) appears to block DA receptors without appreciably affecting noradrenergic receptors, depressed self-stimulation both at central grey and lateral hypothalamic sites (Liebman and Butcher, 1973; Wauquier and Niemegeers, 1972). On the other hand, apomorphine, a DA receptor stimulant, caused facilitation of self-stimulation responding at low doses, maximum being at 0.63 mg/kg and depression at high doses, maximum being at 1.25 mg/kg (Wauquier and Niemegeers, 1973). In another study (Liebman and Butcher, 1973), apomorphine (0.75 and 1.5 mg/kg) as well as L-DOPA itself (75 and 150 mg/kg together with RO4-4602, a peripheral decarboxylase inhibitor) were shown to reduce self-stimulation respondings that were restored to control levels by doubling the current. Thus, over-or under-stimulation of the striatal DA receptors would produce motor abnormalities that would produce behavioral deficit (Ungerstedt, 1971). At the present stage of our knowledge, it appears that in addition to the noradrenergic system, integrity of dopaminergic system appears to be essential for the behavioral expression of certain motivational processes as in self-stimulation. It is possible that a certain ratio between the two catecholamines, NE and DA, needs to be maintained for proper functioning of the systems involved.

(iii) Role of Cholinergic Mechanism

Stark and Boyd (1963) showed that administration of physostigmine, an anticholinesterase agent that can pass through the blood-brain barrier, caused inhibition of self-stimulation in dogs with electrodes implanted in the mammillary region of the hypothalamus. On the other hand, a quaternary ammonium anticholinesterase agent, neostigmine, that cannot cross the blood-brain barrier, failed to show such effect. The inhibitory effect of physostigmine on self-stimulation could be antagonized by a tertiary ammonium anticholinergic alkaloid, atropine, but not by its quaternary ammonium derivative, methyl atropine. This finding was further substantiated in rats with electrodes implanted at various loci in the brain (Jung and Boyd, 1966).

Subsequent investigations (Domino and Olds, 1968, 1972; Olds and Domino, 1969a,b; Olds, 1970, 1972) have also corroborated a cholinergic depression of self-stimulation behavior in rats with respect to physostigmine and arecoline and antagonism to such depressants by anticholinergic agents. Physostigmine-induced depression of self-stimulation behavior could be correlated with a decrease in brain acetylcholinesterase (AChE) activity and resultant increase in brain ACh; an equimolecular dose of neostigmine that failed to cause a change in the concentrations of brain ACh or AChE activity caused less depression (Domino and Olds, 1968). On the other hand, scopolamine (2 mg/kg) caused a significant decrease in brain ACh. During self-stimulation that also caused a reduction in brain ACh, treatment with scopolamine showed a trend for further reduction in brain ACh, although not statistically significant (Domino and Olds, 1972). Neostigmine-induced behavioral depression could be antagonized to some extent by methylscopolamine but not by scopolamine, showing that this depression was due to a peripheral mechanism (Domino and Olds, 1968; Pradhan and Kamat, 1972).

The anticholinergic agents, e.g., atropine, scopolamine, Ditran (JB 329) and JB 336 not only antagonized the cholinergically induced depression of self-stimulation responding, but they themselves caused facilitation of this behavior (Pradhan and Kamat, 1972, 1973). Such effects of anticholinergics were marked, especially when the baseline rate of responding and the doses of the drugs were low. Methylscopolamine failed to produce a consistent effect at comparable doses. Thus, it was evident from these studies that a central _m_-cholinergic (muscarinic) mechanism appears to play an inhibitory role on self-stimulation behavior.

Central nicotinic or _n_-cholinergic mechanism also showed some effects on self-stimulation responding. Olds and Domino (1969a) reported that nicotine produced inconsistent biphasic effects such as initial depression sometimes followed by facilitation. Pradhan and Bowling (1971) using various methods for generating different baseline rates of responding, demonstrated a rate-dependent effect of nicotine. Facilitation of responding was observed at 37.5 μg/kg and higher doses (up to 400 μg/kg used) of nicotine in rats with low response rates. In rats with high response rates, nicotine had very little effect or even caused depression. However, when the rates were lowered in such rats by reducing current intensity or after prolonged lever-pressing or administration of an optimum dose of phenobarbital (10-25 mg/kg) or pentobarbital (15 mg/kg), a facilitatory effect of nicotine could be observed. It counteracted the depressant effect of barbiturates on self-stimulation. Compared in the same rats, the effect of nicotine resembled very closely that of amphetamine in potency as well as in the pattern of activity. Facilitation by nicotine was reduced or blocked by mecamylamine, a tertiary ammonium ganglion blocking agent, and could not be observed in rats pretreated with reserpine 24 hours earlier. It was proposed that nicotine by acting on a central _n_-cholinergic receptor, may cause release of NE which in turn would produce the facilitatory effect on self-stimulation.

(iv) Role of Serotonergic Mechanism

5-HT also plays some role in self-stimulation behavior. Stark _et al_. (1964) used a 5-HT antagonist as well as drugs that alter the brain levels of 5-HT, and also catecholamines to modify self-stimulation responding in dogs. Their data, although not conclusive, suggested a role of 5-HT in this behavior. Use of _p_-chlorophenylalanine (PCPA), an inhibitor of tryptophan hydroxylase, resulted in diverse effects on this behavior, such as inhibition (Margules, 1969; Gibson _et al_., 1970; Stark _et al_., 1970), no effect (Black and Cooper, 1970; Cooper _et al_., 1971), and facilitation (Blum and Geller, 1969; Poschel and Ninteman, 1971). It was further observed that PCPA tended to suppress self-stimulation shortly after administration, but facilitated the same after 3-7 days.

On the other hand, treatment with 5-hydroxytryptophan (5-HTP), a precursor of 5-HT, was shown to depress self-stimulation at a high (300 mg/kg) dose and to stimulate it at smaller (5-10 mg/kg) doses (Poschel and Ninteman, 1968). It was suggested that the excitatory effect might be due to release of NE from its storage sites in the brain (Brodie *et al*., 1966).

In our laboratory (Bose *et al*., 1974), 5-HTP (28, 57 and 115 mg/kg, i.p.) was shown to cause a dose-dependent decrease (32, 57 and 66%, respectively) in self-stimulation responding in rats, whereas other amino acids (*e.g*., glycine, glutamic acid) or the vehicle had negligible effects. A similar decrease although slightly more, but insignificant, was also observed when 5-HTP was given in combination with RO4-4602, a peripheral decarboxylase inhibitor. Concomitant with the decrease in responding, there was a significant increase in 5-HT contents of the various areas of the brain in the treated rats; the NE contents showed only a slight decrease. Thus, an inhibitory role of brain 5-HT in self-stimulation behavior could be demonstrated.

III. Interaction and Balance Among Neurotransmitters in Self-Stimulation

On the basis of available information, existence of interaction and balance between neurotransmitters involved in self-stimulation can be discussed from three different standpoints: neuroanatomical, neurochemical and neuropharmacological.

(i) Neuroanatomical

It is generally considered that during self-stimulation behavior, noradrenergic or dopaminergic neurons are electrically stimulated in the reinforcing brain areas through the implanted electrode. Microneuroanatomical study of many of these areas shows that neurons containing other neurotransmitters may also be involved during such stimulation process. Thus, the medial forebrain bundle-lateral hypothalamic area that is known to be the most prominent reinforcing site has been demonstrated by fluorescence histochemical technique (Andén *et al*., 1966) to contain not only the noradrenergic and dopaminergic neurons, but also serotonergic fibers. Moreover, by utilizing AChE staining technique, Shute (1970) has demonstrated an ascending cholinergic reticular system; in rats and also in cats the majority of the fibers of this system travel to globus pallidus and lateral preoptic area by the medial forebrain bundle via lateral hypothalamus.

Tracing these noradrenergic and dopaminergic tracts backwards to their respective origins, it was demonstrated that electrical stimulation of the locus coeruleus in the rostral pons and that of the interpeduncular nucleus (IPN) in the mesencephalon are both reinforcing (Crow, 1972a, Crow et al., 1972). Furthermore, IPN has been demonstrated to contain very large amounts of choline acetylase (Lewis et al., 1967) and AChE-containing neurons that appear to connect with those of the ventral tegmental pathway of the ascending cholinergic reticular system (Lewis and Shute, 1967; Shute and Lewis, 1967). Similar linkage of the central cholinergic system to many other reward areas may also exist. Because of such close association of neuronal systems containing different transmitters in and around the reward areas, there is a strong possibility of more than one of these systems being affected during self-stimulation. Simultaneous stimulation of multiple systems to varying degrees in a particular reward area generates the pattern characteristic for the site.

(ii) Neurochemical

The neuroanatomical interrelation between different amine-containing neurons can also be correlated to some extent with the neurochemical changes during self-stimulation. By perfusing the hypothalamus and the amygdala of unanesthetized rats through push-pull cannulae, Stein and Wise (1969) demonstrated that NE can be released at the central synapses by rewarding electrical stimulation of the medial forebrain bundle and also by amphetamine. Release of NE and DA was also demonstrated in another way by assessing the reduction of histochemical fluorescence in rats pretreated with amine synthesis inhibitors (e.g., α-methyl p-tyrosine or FLA-63) following electrical stimulation of the central monoamine pathways with stimulation parameters similar to those used in their self-stimulation experiments (Arbuthnott et al., 1970). Such stimulation of noradrenergic and dopaminergic sites was effective in reducing amine-specific fluorescence in the areas of distribution of respective nerve terminals, suggesting release of the transmitters at these locations. On the other hand, Domino and Olds (1972) have demonstrated that brain ACh was reduced during self-stimulation. d-Amphetamine (2 mg/kg) and scopolamine (2 mg/kg) caused significant decrease of brain

ACh in animals not allowed to self-stimulate. Self-stimulation responding in rats treated with these drugs further reduced the brain ACh. Mechanism of such decrease of ACh content is not clear. On the basis of assumption that the stimulation-induced decrease of the contents of NE and DA in the respective neurons is an index of their release, as in the previous experiment (Arbuthnott *et al.*, 1970), it is probable that ACh may also be released during self-stimulation leading to decrease in its content in the brain. However, other possibilities such as decreased formation cannot be ruled out. Whatever may be the mechanism of its decrease, ACh appears to be involved in the chemodynamics of self-stimulation in addition to NE and DA. Moreover, the metabolism of ACh during self-stimulation also appears to be modified by drugs affecting both cholinergic and catecholaminergic mechanisms. Responding can be facilitated by drugs by modifying the proportion of release of various transmitters with preponderance of excitatory ones or by blocking the action of inhibitory ones. Such modification of release of different transmitters during self-stimulation or its pharmacological manipulation appears to be concerted and balanced and not isolated events.

(iii) Neuropharmacological

Self-stimulation responding is inhibited by cholinergic agents, *e.g.*, physostigmine. Anticholinergic agents such as scopolamine not only antagonize the effect of cholinergic agents, but also facilitate self-stimulation responding by themselves (Pradhan and Kamat, 1972, 1973). To explain this, it was proposed that during self-stimulation of certain reward areas, as in the hypothalamus, both noradrenergic excitatory (go) and the cholinergic inhibitory (no-go) systems are stimulated. Self-stimulation responding is dependent upon the balance between the activities of these systems. Anticholinergic agents enhance the responding by blocking the inhibitory cholinergic responses (figure 1-D,E).

When scopolamine was administered prior to physostigmine, it not only antagonized the inhibitory effect of the latter, but further enhanced the responding in most of the subjects, particularly those with low baseline rates (Pradhan and Kamat, 1972). This enhancement can be explained by presuming that as in the peripheral nervous system, there are both muscarinic and nicotinic cholinergic receptors in the brain and, furthermore, the nicotinic receptors are connected with both excitatory noradrenergic (figure 1-C) and inhibitory cholinergic (figure 1-D)

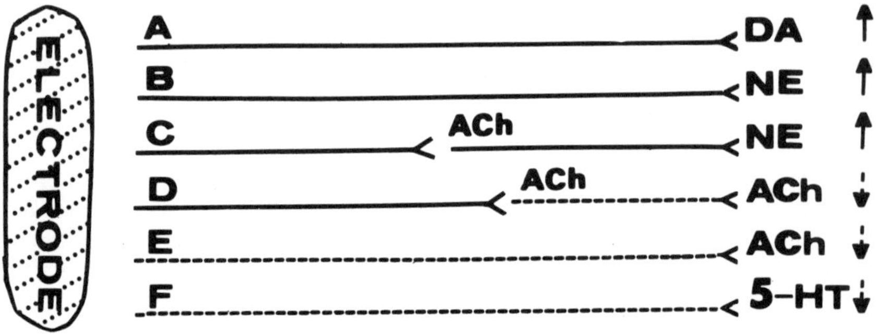

Fig. 1. Possible involvement of neuronal systems containing different transmitters during the self-stimulation behavior. A, dopaminergic (DA); B, noradrenergic (NE); C, n-cholinergic with noradrenergic; D, n- and m-cholinergic; E, m-cholinergic; F, serotonergic (5-HT). Stimulation of respective neurons causes facilitation (↑) or depression (↓) of behavior.

systems. An anticholinesterase agent like physostigmine would cause inhibition by increasing the concentration of ACh, not only at the terminal of the muscarinic neurons, but also at the nicotinic receptor site of the muscarinic neurons and cause facilitation by increasing the concentration of ACh at the nicotinic receptor site of the noradrenergic neurons (figure 1-C). Scopolamine, given in combination with physostigmine, blocked the inhibitory effects of the latter as well as unmasked the noradrenergic facilitation (figure 1-B), including that induced cholinergically by the anticholinesterase (figure 1-C).

This view can be further supported by analyzing the action of nicotine which causes facilitation of self-stimulation responding, particularly at low baseline rates. The facilitatory action of nicotine can be prevented by preadministration of reserpine showing that probably biogenic amines, particularly NE, are involved (Pradhan and Bowling, 1971). On the other hand, further enhancement of nicotine-induced facilitation was observed in about 60% of the animals, when scopolamine was administered in combination, showing that nicotine also stimulates cholinergic as well as noradrenergic neurons (Pradhan and Kamat, 1972).

When self-stimulation is reduced following preadministration with reserpine, scopolamine-induced facilitation of self-stimulation can be demonstrated even more clearly (Pradhan, unpublished data). Reserpine depletes NE, DA, 5-HT and histamine and causes a slight increase or no effect on brain ACh content. This causes a disturbance in the balance between various neurotransmitters, resulting in cholinergic preponderance. Following reserpine treatment, self-stimulation responding is reduced due to both catecholaminergic deficiency and cholinergic preponderance. Scopolamine enhances the responding rate more markedly by blocking the inhibitory muscarinic cholinergic effects.

IV. Summary and Conclusions

Self-stimulation behavior is facilitated by NE and probably DA and inhibited by ACh and 5-HT. It is modulated by their overall involvement and maintained through adrenergic preponderance. It appears that during self-stimulation there is not only an increase in the effective concentrations of facilitatory neurotransmitters like NE and DA, but also a decrease in inhibitory transmitters like ACh and 5-HT at the receptor sites with overall preponderance of the facilitatory ones. The relative proportion of the transmitters involved, rather than the concentration of any individual one, determines the behavioral activity. Drugs and procedures modify self-stimulation behavior by upsetting the balance through modification of the metabolism or activity of one or more components of this multitransmitter system. There are many drugs that affect the metabolism of more than one neurotransmitter system. In addition to the examples cited earlier, the effects of L-DOPA need to be emphasized. Besides increasing the concentrations of DA and NE, L-DOPA also affects ACh content. Thus, in rabbits L-DOPA given i.p. restored to normal levels the striatal ACh content which was decreased following administration of reserpine (Barbeau, 1972). Furthermore, L-DOPA blocks the chlorpromazine-induced decrease in striatal ACh. On the other hand, DA receptor stimulants such as apomorphine and trivastal increase striatal ACh concentration (Sethy and Van Woert, 1974).

In self-stimulation behavior, methodological complexities present some difficulties in proper evaluation of a drug effect, particularly with respect to electrode sites, many of which are related to local distributions of neurotransmitters and pattern of their balance. Most of the studies with drugs reported here have been conducted with placement of the electrode at a single intracranial site, the posterior lateral hypothalamus being the most common. The other sites used include ventromedial and anterior hypothalamus, ventral tegmentum, septum, etc. While there may not be such difficulty in evaluating the effect of a drug with respect to a particular electrode site, the effects of the same drug may vary with respect to different reward areas in the same animal. Furthermore, stimulation of certain areas, e.g., dorso-medial tegmentum, would elicit aversive response. Others may show mixed reactions, reinforcing and aversive (Crow, 1972a,b, 1973; Olds and Travis, 1960; Phillips and Fibiger, 1973; Pradhan and Bowling, 1971). A great deal of these variations may be ascribed to the difference in the local distribution of neurotransmitter - containing neurons.

Evaluation of balance in self-stimulation, as also in many other behaviors, becomes complicated if simultaneous consideration is directed toward the underlying brain systems involved in such behavior. Hypothalamic stimulation has the capability of exciting the substrates of a number of species-specific responses ("fixed action patterns"). Discharging the sensitized or excited substrate is reinforcing and it can provide the motivation to engage in instrumental behavior. The "built-in" characteristics of the individual animals interacting with the modulating inputs from the environment are the major determinants of responses that are elicited (Valenstein, 1970). Furthermore, while proper integrity and efficiency of the motor system involving pyramidal and extrapyramidal tracts may be necessary for "behavioral expression" in the form of specific responding, much more extensive and far more important will be the underlying "behavioral preparation" subsequent to hypothalamic stimulation that would involve, in addition to the reinforcement system, multiple substrates for motivation, drive, learning and memory. Each of these substrates can be modulated by a number of transmitters. Furthermore, the transmitters affecting the reinforcement system will also affect the other related systems, particularly the motor mechanism. Therefore, proper functioning of the reinforcement system necessitates an appropriate balance of the transmitters related not only to this system, but also to the motor and other systems.

A functional system that is modulated by multiple neurotransmitters with appropriate balance between them will be expected to meet at least the following criteria: 1) Among the involved transmitters each of which must satisfy all the necessary criteria for a neurotransmitter, one or more must have opposing action(s) with respect to that of others. ii) The functional state of the system would be determined by the algebraic sum of the opposing actions of the transmitters with a probable relative preponderance of one or more of the components. iii) Alteration of effect of any one of the components induced pathologically or experimentally would cause alteration of one or more of the remaining components (through intervention of a regulating system) in an attempt to maintain homeostasis of the functional system. iv) In case of deficiency induced in a component, restoration towards functional normalization may be achieved by removal of such deficiency by neurochemical, neuropharmacological or other means.

Critical evidences to fulfill some of the criteria, particularly the third one, are not adequate in self-stimulation, as in many other behavior and CNS functions. However, automatic mechanism to maintain homeostasis may not exist in many functional systems. Currently available data have been collected by different investigators separately with respect to different transmitters. To fulfill the criteria of balance adequately, it will be necessary to simultaneously investigate the multiple transmitters involved in this behavior with respect to both synthesis and contents. Until such data are available, present information can be considered as strongly indicative of balance of the neurotransmitters in this behavior.

References

Andén, N.E., Dahlström, A., Fuxe, K., Larsson, K., Olson, L. and Ungerstedt, U.: Ascending monoamine neurons to the telencephalon and diencephalon. Acta Physiol. Scand. 67: 313-326, 1966.

Andén, N.E., Butcher, S.G., Corrodi, H., Fuxe, K. and Ungerstedt, U.: Receptor activity and turnover of dopamine and noradrenaline after neuroleptics. Eur. J. Pharmacol. 11: 303-314, 1970.

Arbuthnott, G.W., Crow, T.J., Fuxe, K., Olson, L. and Ungerstedt, U.: Depletion of catecholamines in vivo induced by electrical stimulation of central monoamine pathways. Brain. Res. 24: 471-483, 1970.

Bailey, P.T., Kamat, K. and Pradhan, S.N.: Effects of adrenergic blocking agents on self-stimulation in rats. Fed. Proc. 31: 573, 1972.

Barbeau, A.: Role of dopamine in the nervous system. Monogram in Human Genetics, 6: 114-136, 1972.

Black, W.C. and Cooper, B.R.: Reduction of electrically-rewarded behavior by interference with monoamine synthesis. Physiol. Behav. 5: 1405-1409, 1970.

Blum, K. and Geller, I.: Facilitation of brain stimulation with para-chlorophenylalanine. Fed. Proc. 28: 794, 1969.

Bose, S., Bailey, P.T., Thoa, N.B. and Pradhan, S.N.: Effects of 5-hydroxytryptophane on self-stimulation in rats. Psychopharmacologia 36: 255-262, 1974.

Breese, G.R., Howard, J.L. and Leahy, J.P.: Effects of 6-hydroxy-dopamine on electrical self-stimulation of the brain. Brit. J. Pharmacol. 43: 255-257, 1971.

Brodie, B.B., Spector, S. and Shore, P.A.: Interaction of drugs with norepinephrine in the brain. Pharmacol. Rev. 11: 548-564, 1959.

Brodie, B.B., Comer, M.S., Costa, E. and Dlabac, A.: The role of brain serotonin in the mechanism of the central action of reserpine. J. Pharmacol. Exp. Ther. 152: 340-349, 1966.

Canfield, D.R., Antelman, S.M., Lippa, A.S. and Fisher, A.E.: Amphetamine-induced alteration of biogenic amines and self-stimulation. Fed. Proc. 32: 754, 1973.

Carlsson, A.: Functional significance of drug-induced changes in brain monoamine levels. Progr. Brain Res. 8: 9-27, 1964.

Carlton, P.L.: Augmentation of the behavioral effects of amphetamine by scopolamine. Psychopharmacologia 2: 377-380, 1961.

Carlton, P.L. and Didamo, P.: Augmentation of the behavioral effects of amphetamine by atropine. J. Pharmacol. Exp. Ther. 132: 91-96, 1961.

Cooper, B.R., Black, W.C. and Paolino, R.M.: Decreased septal-forebrain and lateral hypothalamic reward after alpha methyl-p-tyrosine. Physiol. Behav. 6: 425-429, 1971.

Crow, T.J.: Mode of enhancement of self-stimulation in rats by methamphetamine. Nature 224: 709-710, 1969.

Crow, T.J.: Enhancement by cocaine of intracranial self-stimulation in the rat. Life Sci. 9: 375-381, 1970.

Crow, T.J.: A map of the rat mesencephalon for electrical self-stimulation. Brain Res. 36: 265-273, 1972a.

Crow, T.J.: Catecholamine-containing neurones and electrical self-stimulation. I. Review of some data. Psychol. Med. 2: 414-421, 1972b.

Crow, T.J.: Catecholamine-containing neurones and electrical self-stimulation. 2. A theoretical interpretation and some psychiatric implications. Psychol. Med. 3: 66-73, 1973.

Crow, T.J., Spear, P.J. and Arbuthnott, G.W.: Intracranial self-stimulation with electrodes in the region of the locus coeruleus. Brain Res. 36: 275-287, 1972.

Dahlström, A. and Fuxe, K.: Evidence for the existence of monoamine-containing neurons in the central nervous system. Acta Physiol. Scand. 62: Suppl. 232, 1-55, 1965.

Domino, E.F. and Olds, M.E.: Cholinergic inhibition of self-stimulation behavior. J. Pharmacol. Exp. Ther. 164: 202-211, 1968.

Domino, E.F. and Olds, M.E.: Effects of d-amphetamine, scopolamine, chlordiazepoxide and diphenylhydantoin on self-stimulation behavior and brain acetylcholine. Psychopharmacologia 23: 1-16, 1972.

Dresse, A.: Influence de 15 neuroleptiques (butyrophénones et phenothiazines) sur les variations de la teneur du cerveau en noradrénaline et l'activité du rat dans le test d'autostimulation. Arch. int. Pharmacodyn. 159: 353-365, 1966a.

Dresse, A.: Importance du systeme mesencephalo-telencephalique noradrenergique comme substratum anatomique du comportement d'autostimulation. Life Sci. 5: 1003-1014, 1966b.

Fog, R.L.: Stereotyped and non-stereotyped behavior in rats induced by various stimulant drugs. Psychopharmacologia 14: 299-304, 1969.

Gibson, S., McGeer, E.G. and McGeer, P.L.: Effect of selective inhibitor of tyrosine and tryptophane hydroxylase on self-stimulation in the rat. Exp. Neurol. 27: 283-290, 1970.

Glisson, S.N., Karczmar, A.G. and Barnes, L.: Cholinergic effects on adrenergic neurotransmitters in rabbit brain parts. Neuropharmacol. 11: 465-477, 1972.

Glowinski, J.: Release of monoamines in the central nervous system. In New Aspects of Storage and Release Mechanisms of Catecholamines, ed. by H.J. Schümann and G. Kroneberg, pp. 237-248, Springer-Verlag, New York, 1970.

Hess, W.R.: Diencephalon: Autonomic and Extrapyramidal Functions. Monogr. Biol. Med. 3, New York, Grune and Stratton, 1954.

Ho, A.K.S., Singer, G. and Gershon, S.: Biochemical evidence of adrenergic interaction with cholinergic function in the central nervous system of the rat. Psychopharmacologia 21: 238-246, 1971.

Ho, A.K.S., and Loh, H.H.: Evidence of adrenergic-cholinergic interaction in the central nervous system. II. Dopamine and its analogues. Eur. J. Pharmacol. 19: 145-150, 1972.

Izquierdo, J.A.: Cholinergic mechanism - monoamines relation in certain brain structures. Progress in Drug Research. 16: 335-363, 1972.

Janssen, P.A.J., Niemegeers, C.J.E., Schellebens, K.H.L., Dresse, A., Lenaerts, F.M., Pinchard, A., Schaper, W.K.A., Van Nueten, J.M. and Verbruggen, F.J.: Pimozide, a chemically novel, highly potent and orally long-acting neuroleptic drugs. I. The comparative pharmacology of pimozide, haloperidol, and chlorpromazine. Arzeimittel-Forsch. 18: 261-279, 1968.

Jung, O.H. and Boyd, E.S.: Effects of cholinergic drugs on self-stimulation response rates in rats. Am. J. Physiol. 210: 432-434, 1966.

Lewis, P.R. and Shute, C.C.D.: The cholinergic limbic system: Projections to hippocampal formation, medial cortex, nuclei of the ascending cholinergic reticular system, and the subfornical organ and supraoptic crest. Brain 90: 520-539, 1967.

Lewis, P.R., Shute, C.C.D. and Silver, A.: Confirmation from choline acetylase analyses of a massive cholinergic innervation to the rat hippocampus. J. Physiol. 191: 215-224, 1967.

Liebman, J.M. and Butcher, L.L.: Effects on self-stimulation behavior of drugs influencing dopaminergic neurotransmission mechanism. Naunyn-Schmiedeberg Arch. Pharmacol. 277: 305-318, 1973.

Lomax, P., Foster, R.S. and Kirkpatrick, W.E.: Cholinergic and adrenergic interactions in the thermoregulatory center of the rat. Brain Res. 15: 431-438, 1969.

Margules, D.L.: Noradrenergic synapses for the suppression of feeding behavior. Life Sci. 8: 693-704, 1969.

Mennear, J.H.: Interactions between central cholinergic agents and amphetamine in mice. Psychopharmacologia 7: 107-114, 1965.

Munkvad, I., Pakkenberg, H. and Randrup, A.: Aminergic systems in basal ganglia associated with stereotyped hyperactive behavior and catalepsy. Brain Behav. Evol. 1: 89-100, 1968.

Olds, J.: Self-stimulation of the brain. Science 127: 315-324, 1958.

Olds, J.: Hypothalamic substrates of reward. Physiol. Rev. 42: 554-604, 1962.

Olds, J., Killam, F.F. and Bach-Y-Rita, P.: Self-stimulation of the brain used as screening method for tranquilizing drugs. Science 124: 265-266, 1956.

Olds, J. and Travis, R.P.: Effects of chlorpromazine, meprobamate, pentobarbital and morphine on self-stimulation. J. Pharmacol. Exp. Ther. 128: 397-404, 1960.

Olds, M.E.: Comparative effects of amphetamine, scopolamine, chlordiazepoxide and diphenylhydantoin on operant and extinction behavior with brain stimulation and food reward. Neuropharmacol. 9: 519-532, 1970.

Olds, M.E.: Alterations by centrally acting drugs of the suppression of self-stimulation behavior in the rat by tetrabenazine, physostigmine, chlorpromazine and pentobarbital. Psychopharmacologia 25: 299-314, 1972.

Olds, M.E. and Domino, E.F.: Comparison of muscarinic and nicotinic cholinergic agonists on self-stimulation behavior. J. Pharmacol. Exp. Ther. 166: 189-204, 1969a.

Olds, M.E. and Domino, E.F.: Differential effects of cholinergic agonists on self-stimulation and escape behavior. J. Pharmacol. Exp. Ther. 170: 157-167, 1969b.

Philippu, A.: Release of catecholamines from the hypothalamus by drugs and electrical stimulation. In New Aspects of Storage and Release Mechanisms of Catecholamines, ed. by H.J. Schümann and G. Kroneberg, pp. 258-267, Springer-Verlag, New York, 1970.

Phillips, A.G. and Fibiger, H.C.: Dopaminergic and noradrenergic substrates of positive reinforcement: Differential effects of d- and l-amphetamine. Science 179: 575-577, 1973.

Poschel, B.P.H. and Ninteman, F.W.: Norepinephrine: A possible excitatory neurohormone of the reward system. Life Sci. 10: 782-788, 1963.

Poschel, B.P.H. and Ninteman, F.W.: Excitatory effects of monoamine oxidase inhibitors on the reward system of the brain. Life Sci. 3: 903-910, 1964.

Poschel, B.P.H. and Ninteman, F.W.: Hypothalamic self-stimulation: Its suppression by blockade of norepinephrine biosynthesis and its reinstatement by methamphetamine. Life Sci. 5: 11-16, 1966.

Poschel, B.P.H. and Ninteman, F.W.: Excitatory effects of 5-HTP on intracranial self-stimulation following MAO blockade. Life Sci. 7: 317-323, 1968.

Poschel, B.P.H. and Ninteman, F.W.: Intracranial reward and the forebrain's serotonergic mechanism: Studies employing para-chlorophenylalanine and para-chloroamphetamine. Physiol. Behav. 7: 39-46, 1971.

Pradhan, S.N. and Bowling, C.: Effects of nicotine on self-stimulation in rats. J. Pharmacol. Exp. Ther. 176: 229-243, 1971.

Pradhan, S.N. and Dutta, S.N.: Central cholinergic mechanism and behavior. Intern. Rev. Neurobiol. 14: 173-231, 1971.

Pradhan, S.N. and Kamat, K.A.: Action and interactions of cholinergic agonists and antagonists on self-stimulation. Arch. Int. Pharmacodyn. 196: 321-329, 1972.

Pradhan, S.N. and Kamat, K.A.: Effects of anticholinergic agents on self-stimulation. Arch. Int. Pharmacodyn. 201: 16-24, 1973.

Ray, O.S. and Bivens, L.W.: Anticholinergic potentiation of amphetamine: Reinforcement schedule effects. Arch. Int. Pharmacodyn. 172: 414-420, 1968.

Rech, R., Borys, H. and Moore, K.: Alterations in behavior and brain catecholamine levels in rats treated with α-methyl-tyrosine. J. Pharmacol. Exp. Ther. 153: 412-419, 1966.

Roll, S.K.: Intracranial self-stimulation and wakefulness: Effect of manipulating ambient brain catecholamines. Science 168: 1370-1372, 1970.

Sethy, V.H. and Van Woert, M.H.: Dopamine receptors and striatal acetylcholine concentration. Fed. Proc. 33: 552, 1974.

Shute, C.C.D. and Lewis, P.R.: The ascending cholinergic reticular system: Neocortical, olfactory and subcortical projections. Brain 90: 497-519, 1967.

Shute, C.C.D.: Distribution of cholinesterase and cholinergic pathways. In The Hypothalamus, ed. by L. Martini, M. Motta and F. Fraschini, pp. 167-179, Academic Press, New York, 1970.

Stark, P. and Boyd, E.S.: Effects of cholinergic drugs on hypothalamic self-stimulation response rates in dogs. Am. J. Physiol. 205: 745-748, 1963.

Stark, P., Boyd, E.S. and Fuller, W.R.: A possible role of serotonin in hypothalamic self-stimulation in dogs. J. Pharmacol. Exp. Ther. 146: 147-153, 1964.

Stark, P., Turk, J.A., Redman, C.E. and Henderson, H.K.: Sensitivity and specificity of positive reinforcing areas to neurosedatives, antidepressants and stimulants. J. Pharmacol. Exp. Ther. 166: 163-169, 1969.

Stark, P., Fuller, R.W., Hartley, L.W., Schaffer, R.J. and Turk, J.A.: Dissociation of the effects of p-chlorophenylalanine on self-stimulation and on brain serotonin. Life Sci. 9: 41-48, 1970.

Stein, L.: Stimulation of the brain and the central stimulant action of amphetamine. Fed. Proc. 23: 836-850, 1964.

Stein, L.: Chemistry of reward and punishment. In Psychopharmacology, ed. by D.H. Efron, J.O. Cole, J. Levine, and J.R. Wittenborn, pp. 105-123, USPHS Publication No. 1836, U.S. Government Printing Office, Washington, D.C., 1968.

Stein, L. and Seifter, J.: Possible mode of antidepressant action of imipramine. Science 134: 286-287, 1961.

Stein, L. and Wise, C.D.: Release of norepinephrine from hypothalamus and amygdala by rewarding medial forebrain bundle stimulation and amphetamine. J. Comp. Physiol. Psychol. 67: 189-198, 1969.

Stein, L. and Wise, C.D.: Possible etiology of schizophrenia: Progressive damage to the noradrenergic reward system by 6-hydroxydopamine. Science 171: 1032-1036, 1971.

Ungerstedt, U.: Adipsia and aphagia after 6-hydroxydopamine-induced degeneration of the nigro-striatal dopamine system. Acta Physiol. Scand. Suppl. 367: 95-122, 1971.

Valenstein, E.S.: Stability and plasticity of motivation systems. In The Neurosciences, Second Study Program, ed. by F.O. Schmitt, pp. 207-217, The Rockefeller University Press, New York, 1970.

Wauquier, A. and Niemegeers, C.J.E.: Intracranial self-stimulation in rats as a function of various stimulus parameters. II. Influence of haloperidol, pimozide and pipamperone on medial forebrain stimulation with monopolar electrodes. Psychopharmacologia 27: 191-203, 1972.

Wauquier, A. and Niemegeers, C.J.E.: Intracranial self-stimulation in rats as a function of various stimulus parameters. III. Influence of apomorphine on medial forebrain bundle stimulation with monopolar electrodes. Psychopharmacologia 30: 163-172, 1973.

Wise, C.D. and Stein, L.: Facilitation of brain stimulation by central administration of norepinephrine. Science 163: 299-301, 1969.

Neurotransmitter Balances Regulating Behavior,
edited and published by E.F. Domino and
J.M. Davis, Ann Arbor, © 1975

EVIDENCE OF A CENTRAL NORADRENERGIC DEFICIENCY IN SCHIZOPHRENIA

C. David Wise and Larry Stein
Wyeth Laboratories
Philadelphia, Pennsylvania

Sixty years ago, Bleuler (1911) coined the term "schizophrenia" (a splitting of the mind) to designate a disease in which the integration of behavior and personality is fundamentally disturbed. The mental functions, he noted, "do not combine in a conglomeration of strivings with a unified resultant as they do in a healthy person"; rather, one group of ideas or drives "dominates the personality for a time, while other groups...are 'split-off' and seem either partly or completely impotent."

Purpose is the psychic glue, according to Bleuler's analysis, on which the coherence of behavior and personality depends. In schizophrenia, the association of ideas is not adequately "related and directed by any unifying concept of purpose or goal." As a result, schizophrenic "thinking becomes illogical and often bizarre", while "schizophrenic behavior is marked by a lack of interest, lack of initiative, lack of a definite goal, by inadequate adaptation to the environment."

In the related view of Rado (1962), the crucial defect in schizophrenia is based in the organizing action of pleasure or reward. According to Rado, "schizophrenic disorders may be viewed as so many experiments of Nature, showing what happens to central integration in the person whose pleasure resources are inherently deficient." In general, "absence of sufficient pleasure slows down and hinders psychodynamic integration, as the absence of an essential enzyme slows down or hinders a complex biochemical process."

CENTRAL NORADRENERGIC PATHWAYS FOR REWARD

Research findings in many different fields (Miller, 1957; Olds, 1962; Stein, 1964; Hillarp _et al._, 1966; Wise and Stein, 1969; Kety, 1972a) have identified central noradrenergic (NE) pathways tentatively associated with pleasure or reward and, hence, with the organization and control of goal directed thinking and behavior (Stein, 1968; Stein _et al._, 1972). Recent histochemical work suggests that NE neurons may be organized into 3 main ascending systems (Lindvall and Björklund, 1974). A "dorsal" pathway originates in the locus coeruleus and principally innervates the cerebral cortex and hippocampus, and "ventral" and "periventricular" pathways originate in the reticular formation and central gray matter of the lower brain stem. These latter pathways principally innervate the hypothalamus and limbic system. Brain self-stimulation studies in animals suggest that all 3 NE pathways mediate rewarding effects (Ritter and Stein, 1974; Stein, 1975).

The differentiation or specialization of reward function among the 3 systems has not yet been worked out. However, the innervation of hypothalamus and limbic system by ventral and periventricular pathways suggests their involvement in motivation and affect. The cortical distribution of the dorsal pathway, and the capacity of its neurons for regeneration and new growth -- and hence for reorganization -- suggests an involvement in learning and associative thinking. Thus, if Bleuler's and Rado's concepts of schizophrenia are correct, it would be necessary only to posit a chronic dysfunction of the NE reward system to explain the schizophrenic disorder of affect and derangement of goal-directed thinking and behavior. In our model of the disease (Stein and Wise, 1971), we accordingly have assumed that NE pathways and their rich terminal systems in diencephalon and limbic forebrain are the sites of critical damage.

To evaluate the validity of this idea, Wise and Stein (1973) conducted postmortem studies of enzymes in human brain. Their finding that dopamine-β-hydroxylase (DBH) activity is significantly reduced in schizophrenics' brains is consistent with the suggestion that disturbance or damage to NE (DBH-containing) neurons is etiologically related to the disease.

DOPAMINE-β-HYDROXYLASE IN NORMAL AND SCHIZOPHRENIC BRAIN

Damage to central NE neurons can be estimated by measuring the DBH in various regions of the brain. DBH catalyzes the β-hydroxylation of dopamine (Kaufman and Friedman, 1965), the last step in the biosynthesis of NE, and is "distributed in brain with a regional pattern of activity that parallels levels of norepinephrine" (Axelrod, 1972). Electrolytic or chemical damage to central NE tracts causes similar reductions in brain NE and DBH (Reis and Molinoff, 1972). Indeed, the enzyme is used as a marker in immunofluorescence studies to visualize the NE pathways (Fuxe et al., 1970; Hartman and Udenfriend, 1972). These and other results lead to the conclusion that "in brain, as in the periphery, DBH is intraneuronal and primarily restricted to those nerve cells synthesizing norepinephrine" (Reis and Molinoff, 1972).

As a first approach, we therefore assumed that measurements of DBH in postmortem samples of human brain could serve as an indicator of the integrity of NE systems.

The availability of a specific and sensitive assay enabled us to measure the low concentrations of DBH in brain homogenates (Bonnay _et al._, 1970; Molinoff _et al._, 1970; Molinoff _et al._, 1971). The two-stage assay uses tyramine as a substrate, and is based on the sequential conversion of the octopamine formed by DBH to radioactively labeled synephrine. Full activity of the enzyme is variably reduced in different brain regions by endogenous inhibitors; these are neutralized by dilution and binding with copper. For optimal enzyme activity in each brain region, final copper sulfate concentrations and dilution of homogenates were as follows: pons-medulla, 30 μmol, 1:40; diencephalon, 24 μmol, 1:30, hippocampus, 15 μmol, 1:30. These parameters were determined separately for schizophrenic and normal brain and did not differ.

Brain specimens were obtained from 8 male and 10 female patients with a diagnosis of chronic schizophrenia who died at Norristown State Hospital, Norristown, Pennsylvania, at a mean age of 71.2 years (range, 45 to 97). The average duration of hospitalization of these patients was 34.4 years (range, 5 to 60). Control material was obtained through the Medical Examiner's Office, New York City, from 6 male and 6 female subjects with no known psychiatric history, who died suddenly in accidents or from heart attacks at an average age of 57.2 years (range, 26 to 80). Care was taken to exclude drug addicts, alcoholics, and suicides from the control group. Also excluded from statistical analysis was one control with head injury who died after 12 days in coma; at autopsy, anoxic necrosis of the brain was found.

The pons-medulla, diencephalon, and hippocampus were dissected out at autopsy and frozen on dry ice. The brain parts were stored at -15° C in plastic bags for varying periods prior to enzymatic analysis; mean storage time $\pm$ S.D. was 3.3 ± 3.1 months for control specimens and 2.7 ± 1.0 months for schizophrenic specimens. Periodic redeterminations of DBH in several cases revealed that the enzyme was stable under these storage conditions, although reduced activity was observed after storage for more than one year. Autopsies generally were performed after postmortem intervals of several hours at room temperature and 1 to 3 days at 4° C. Intervals between death and autopsy were as follows: 4 controls and 4 schizophrenics were autopsied on day of death; 4 controls and 6 schizophrenics, 1 day after death; 2 controls and 1 schizophrenic, 2 days after death; 1 control and 1 schizophrenic, 3 days after death; 3 schizophrenics, 4 days after death; 2 schizophrenics, 6 days after death; 1 schizophrenic, 8 days after death; and for 1 autopsied control, the time of death was unknown.

To assess the effects of postmortem decomposition on brain DBH, we killed rats with ether and then exposed different groups prior to autopsy to roughly the same conditions of time and temperature as those encountered in our human studies. After 3 hrs at room temperature, DBH was reduced by 27 percent, as illustrated in figure 1. However, storage at 4° C for an additional 1 to 3 days led only to small further decreases in enzyme activity. In a follow-up experiment, the postmortem effects of intervals of up to 24 hrs at room temperature were studied, using rats that had been killed nontraumatically with carbon dioxide. Under these conditions, DBH activity was reduced by only 23 percent under 24 hrs (table 1).

For human assays, 400 mg samples of pons-medulla and diencephalon, and 150 mg samples of hippocampus, were used. To ensure random sampling, a whole brain region was immersed in its plastic bag in liquid nitrogen and then fragmented by hammering. The fragments were sifted and particles 2 to 3.4 mm in diameter were retained. After weighing, the samples were homogenized and assayed for DBH according to the procedure of Molinoff _et al_. (1971). Three samples of particles were analyzed in duplicate on different days for an individual brain region (6 determinations). Diencephalic samples were assayed at 5 different tyramine concentrations. Each diencephalic data point used for statistical analysis thus represents the average of 30 determinations.

There was a significant reduction in DBH activity in the schizophrenic group in all brain regions examined (table 2). The deficits were somewhat larger in rostral regions (diencephalon and hippocampus) where the nerve terminals are localized than in caudal regions (pons-medulla) where the cell bodies are localized. Individual values of diencephalic DBH in the 2 groups were distributed with little overlap (figure 2A); only 3 schizophrenic values fell in the normal range. Significant deficits in diencephalic DBH were found at all tyramine concentrations (figure 2B).

EVALUATION OF DOPAMINE-β-HYDROXYLASE DEFICIT IN SCHIZOPHRENIA: ROLE OF EXTRANEOUS FACTORS

Control experiments were conducted to rule out the possibility that the DBH deficiency resulted from postmortem changes. We matched control and schizophrenic cases for morgue-to-autopsy time and still found a significant group

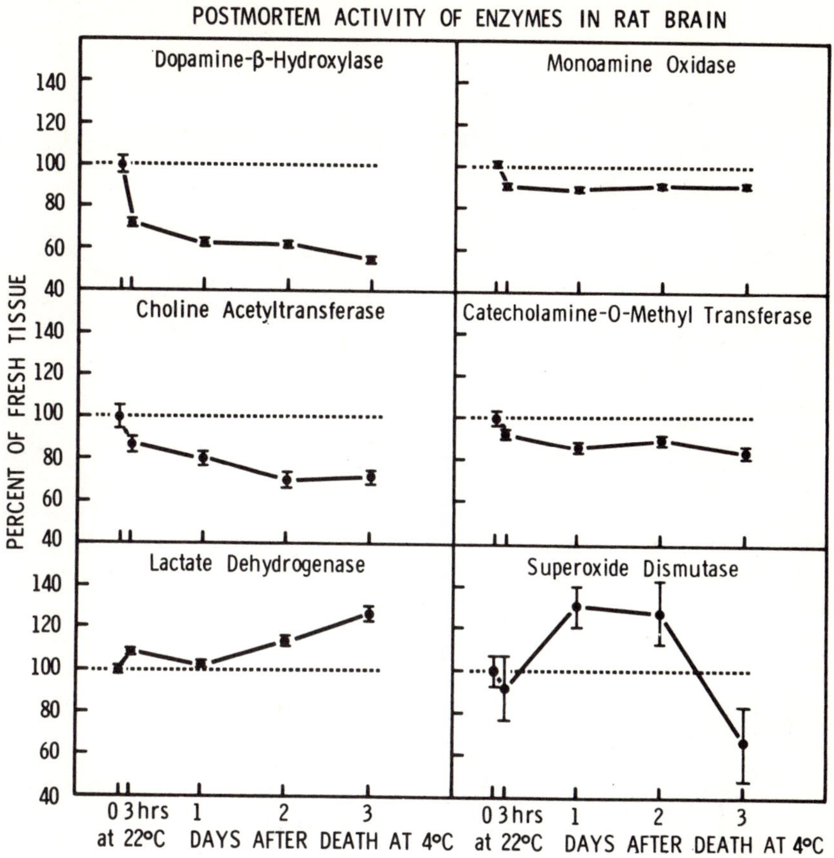

Fig. 1. Postmortem activity of various enzymes in rat brain (whole brain minus neocortex and cerebellum). Groups of 5 rats each were killed with ether and then stored prior to autopsy for different periods of time at 4° C after an initial 3 hr interval at 22° C. Fresh tissue reference groups (dashed lines) were autopsied immediately after death. Absolute values for reference groups were as follows: Dopamine-β-hydroxylase, 27.6 ± 2.0 nmol per g per 20 min; Monoamine oxidase, 6.43 ± 0.06 μmol per g per hr; Choline acetyltransferase, 6.55 ± 3.78 nmol per g per hr; Lactate dehydrogenase, 54.6 ± 1.56 extinction units per g per 120 sec; Superoxide dismutase, 0.48 ± 0.07 arbitrary enzyme units. Bars indicate S.E.

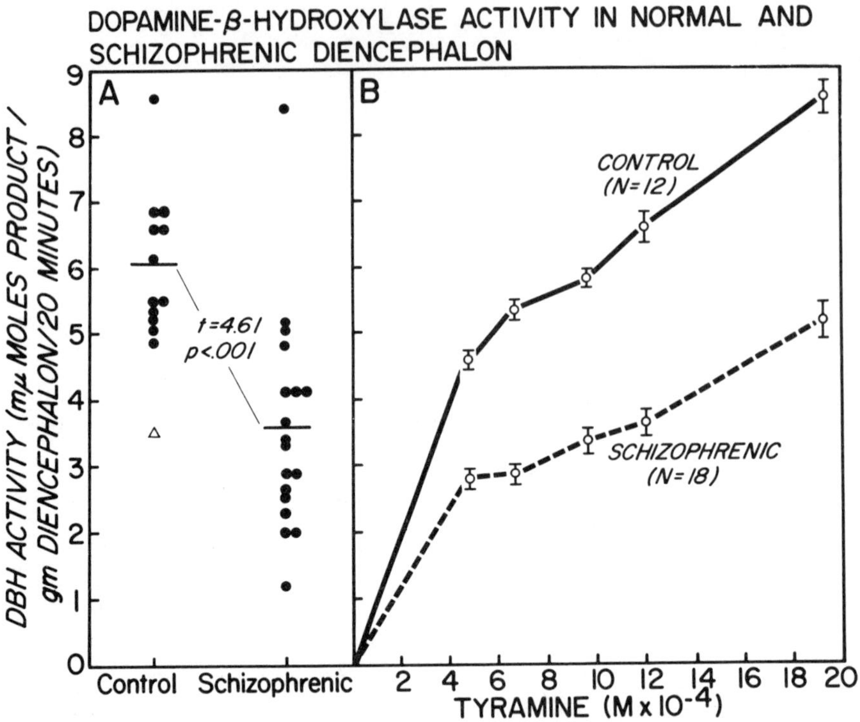

Fig. 2. Dopamine-β-hydroxylase (DBH) activity in postmortem specimens of diencephalon from 18 schizophrenic patients and 12 normal controls. (A) Distributions of individual values of diencephalic DBH. Each point is the average of 30 assays (6 determinations at each of 5 different tyramine concentrations); these values are used for all analyses of diencephalic DBH reported in the text. Horizontal lines indicate means of distributions. Triangle shows DBH activity from a control case which was excluded from statistical analysis because of anoxic necrosis of the brain. The highest value in the schizophrenic group represents the case that had been autopsied 8 days after death. (B) The DBH activity as a function of a substrate concentration. Activity in schizophrenic groups is significantly reduced ($P < .001$) as compared to control group at every concentration of tyramine. Bars indicate S.E. (From Wise and Stein, 1973.)

Table 1

Postmortem deterioration of dopamine-β-hydroxylase (DBH) activity in whole rat brain (minus neocortex and cerebellum)[a]

Storage Time at 22°C (hr)	Mean DBH Activity ± S.E.	% of 0-hr Control
0	24.2 ± 0.96	-
3	22.8 ± 0.80	94.1 ± 3.34
7	17.6 ± 0.59	72.6 ± 2.44
17	19.5 ± 1.72	80.4 ± 7.12
24	18.8 ± 1.06	77.6 ± 4.40

[a]Rats were killed by immersion in carbon dioxide and then stored at room temperature prior to autopsy for the indicated intervals. Enzyme activity is expressed as nmol of octopamine formed per g of tissue per hr. Assay of Molinoff _et al._, 1971.

Table 2

Dopamine-β-hydroxylase in postmortem specimens of brain from 18 schizophrenic patients and 12 controls[a]

Region	Control	Schizophrenic	
	Mean Activity ± S.E.	Mean Activity ± S.E.	Percent of Control
Pons-Medulla	8.86 ± 0.86	6.09 ± 0.61[b]	70.1
Diencephalon	5.83 ± 0.30	3.38 ± 0.39[c]	57.9
Hippocampus	2.87 ± 0.52	1.42 ± 0.38[d]	49.4

[a]Enzyme activity is expressed as nmol per g per 20 min. The concentration of tyramine used in all assays was 9.6×10^{-4} M; S.E., standard error of the mean. From Wise and Stein (1973).
[b]Differs from control, $P < .02$.
[c]Differs from control, $P < .001$.
[d]Differs from control, $P < .05$.

difference ($P < .001$). Furthermore, it is possible that, as a result of unknown factors, the DBH in the schizophrenics' brains deteriorated at a more rapid rate after death than the DBH in normal brain. We therefore plotted the course of deterioration of the enzyme for the 2 groups (figure 3). A difference in the rate of postmortem deterioration would have produced divergent curves. Instead, the 2 curves followed roughly parallel courses and were well separated at all time points, which suggests that the deterioration of DBH was similar in the 2 groups. Indeed, a significant deficit in schizophrenic DBH activity was obtained in a test involving only the 8 cases that had received autopsies on the day of death ($P < .02$).

We next examined the possibility that antipsychotic medications caused the DBH deficiency. Since various phenothiazines had been administered at one time or another to nearly all of our patients, we could not use our human material to determine whether these drugs might inhibit DBH in the brain. We therefore gave rats daily doses (20 mg/kg) of chlorpromazine for prolonged periods. The drug did not inhibit brain DBH even at this high dosage. In fact, after 12 weeks of treatment, a small but statistically reliable increase in enzyme activity was found ($P < .02$, Wise and Stein, 1973).

We next examined the possibility that the greater mean age of the schizophrenic patients contributed to the reduction in DBH. To compare individuals of equivalent age, we again analyzed the data of all normal (N=9) and schizophrenic (N=14) subjects who died between the ages of 45 and 80. Although the mean age of death of these matched subjects was nearly identical (control, 64.1 ± 3.9 years and schizophrenic, 66.9 ± 2.8 years), diencephalic DBH activity was still significantly reduced in the schizophrenic subgroup. The magnitude of the deficit after matching for age was nearly the same as that found originally (age-matched control, 5.89 ± 0.25 and age-matched schizophrenic, 3.96 ± 0.42, $P < .005$).

Differences in the cause of death also fail to explain the enzyme deficit in the schizophrenic group. When this factor was controlled by considering only victims of heart attack (a total of 5 control and 9 schizophrenic cases), there was still a significant reduction in the diencephalic DBH activity of the patients as compared to the controls (control, 5.59 ± 0.30 and schizophrenic, 3.48 ± 0.42, $P < .01$). Furthermore, within the control group, the DBH activity in the diencephalon of the 5 heart attack cases did not differ significantly from that (6.45 ± 0.50) of the 7 accident victims.

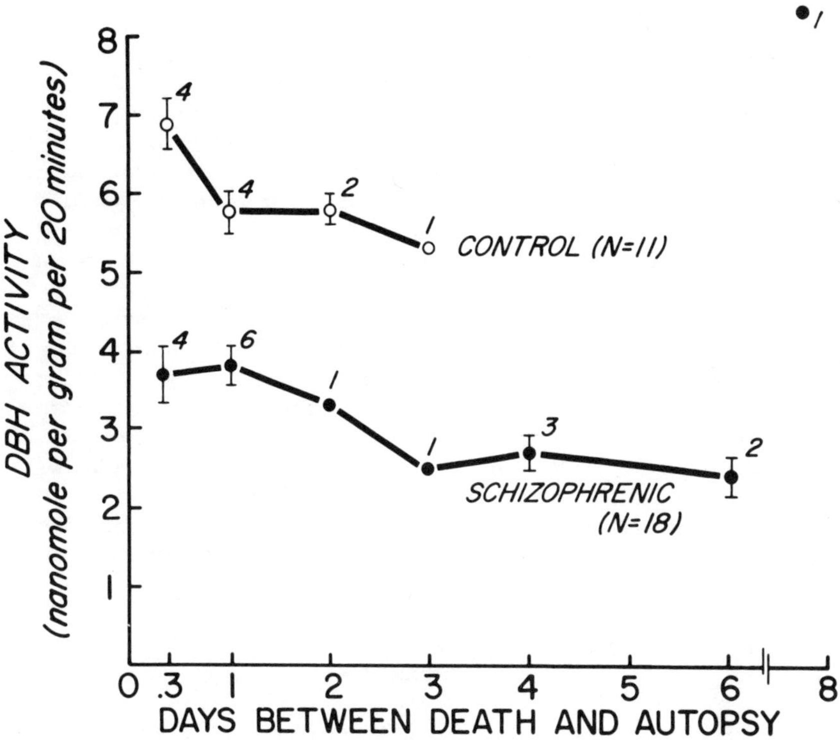

Fig. 3. Postmortem deterioration of dopamine-β-hydroxylase (DBH) in the diencephalon of schizophrenic patients and normal controls. Parallel curves suggest similar rates of deterioration in the two groups. The number of cases of each time point is indicated. Note that the highest value in the schizophrenic group is the case autopsied 8 days after death. Bars indicate standard errors.

Similar DBH deficiencies were found for male and female schizophrenics, consistent with the similar incidence of the disease in the 2 sexes (female control, 6.38 ± 0.58 and male control, 5.80 ± 0.33; female schizophrenic, 3.90 ± 0.48 and male schizophrenic, 3.23 ± 0.48). No relation was found between diencephalic DBH activity and duration of hospitalization (correlation coefficient = .02), although periods of institutionalization in our sample of chronic schizophrenics ranged from 5 to 60 years. Furthermore, the mean DBH of 12 patients hospitalized for more than 30 years (mean hospitalization, 42.9 years; DBH, 3.53 ± 0.56) did not differ significantly from that of 6 patients hospitalized for less than 30 years (mean hospitalization, 17.3 years; DBH, 3.74 ± 0.52). These results do not support the idea that the schizophrenic deficit in DBH is due to hospitalization, but final evaluation of this factor must await further study of nonhospitalized schizophrenics and hospitalized controls.

Some physiochemical properties of diencephalic DBH were examined in normal and schizophrenic subjects. The Michaelis constants (K_m) for tyramine were closely similar and both values were almost identical to that previously obtained from normal human blood serum (table 3).

Table 3

Substrate K_m of dopamine-β-hydroxylase from various tissues

Tissue	Substrate K_m (10^{-4}M Tyramine)
Rat Serum[a]	6.3 ± 0.8
Normal Human Serum[a]	6.5 ± 2.1
Normal Human Adrenal[a]	8.1 ± 1.8
Normal Human Brain	6.7 ± 1.0
Schizophrenic Brain	7.3 ± 1.4

[a]Values from Ross *et al.*, 1972

The K_m values for the ascorbic acid cofactors also were similar in the 2 groups (control, 1.4 x 10^{-4}M ± 0.1, N=2 and schizophrenic, 1.1 x 10^{-4}M ± .03, N=4). Diencephalic

DBH from both groups showed linearity of reaction with respect to dilution and time up to 30 min of incubation. The initial velocity was proportionately lower in the schizophrenic group. Dialysis of control and schizophrenic homogenates for 2 hrs in a 0.005 M tris buffer, pH 5, containing 0.1 percent Triton X-100, did not change DBH activity.

SPECIFICITY OF THE DOPAMINE-β-HYDROXYLASE DEFICIT IN SCHIZOPHRENIA

The foregoing results suggest that the DBH deficiency in schizophrenic patients cannot be attributed to extraneous factors such as postmortem deterioration, drugs, age differences, cause of death, sex, or duration of hospitalization. The deficit in DBH might therefore be associated with the disease itself. If so, then questions arise as to the specificity of the deficit. Are enzymes other than DBH deficient in schizophrenia? Is DBH deficient in mental diseases other than schizophrenia? A satisfactory answer to both questions requires that many enzymes be measured in many different patient groups. In an attempt to provide a preliminary answer to the first question, we assayed 5 enzymes in addition to DBH in normal and schizophrenic brain (Wise *et al.*, 1974).

Lactate dehydrogenase. For an initial comparison with DBH, we were interested in an enzyme that is not specialized for nervous function. Lactate dehydrogenase is a key enzyme in carbohydrate metabolism with a general distribution in the body. Unlike DBH, lactate dehydrogenase in the rat brain does not decline and even may increase in activity for up to 3 days after death (figure 1). The activity of this enzyme was similar in control and schizophrenic specimens (lactate dehydrogenase activity, assayed by a modification [Johnson, 1960] of the method of Kornberg [1955], and expressed as extinction units per 2 min per g of diencephalon: control, 48.3 ± 1.0, N = 12; and schizophrenic, 47.0 ± 1.9, N = 18). This result suggests that grossly nonspecific factors, such as denaturation of brain protein, may be ruled out as explanations of the DBH deficit in the schizophrenic group.

Monoamine oxidase. We next assayed the activity of monoamine oxidase, a major enzyme in the metabolism of the biogenic amines. This enzyme was of particular interest since monoamine oxidase activity in blood platelets has been reported to be markedly reduced in chronic and acute schizophrenics (Murphy and Wyatt, 1972). Furthermore, since nonschizophrenic co-twins of schizophrenic patients also have significantly reduced enzyme activity, it has been suggested that platelet monoamine oxidase may be a genetic marker for vulnerability to schizophrenia (Wyatt et al., 1973).

Brain monoamine oxidase was assayed by the method of Wurtman and Axelrod (1963). In the rat brain, monoamine oxidase is highly stable for up to 3 days after death (figure 1). No differences between normal and schizophrenic enzyme activity were obtained in any brain region, neither in the total sample nor after matching for age (table 4). The discrepancy between these negative results in brain and the earlier findings in platelets may be due to various factors. First, brain monoamine oxidase exists in at least 2 forms, A and B, whereas the platelets contain only form B (Neff et al., 1974). Secondly, most of the brain monoamine oxidase is contained in the glia with only a small fraction in the neurons (Neff, personal communication). Thus, analysis of total brain monoamine oxidase probably would not reveal a schizophrenic deficit in neuronal monoamine oxidase even if such a deficit exists.

Superoxide dismutase. Superoxide dismutase catalyzes the decay of the superoxide anion, a free radical of high biological toxicity. The generation of the superoxide radical by both enzymatic and nonenzymatic oxidations of biological significance and the protective effects of superoxide dismutase have been demonstrated by several investigators (see review, Fridovich, 1972). The superoxide radical has been shown recently to be formed during the autooxidation of 6-hydroxydopamine, and it has been suggested that this radical may mediate the adrenergic nerve terminal degeneration caused by 6-hydroxydopamine (Heikkila and Cohen, 1973). Since a low concentration of superoxide dismutase would increase the susceptibility of neuronal tissue to the superoxide radical, and since we have already speculated that 6-hydroxydopamine or a closely related substance may be involved in schizophrenia (Stein and Wise, 1971), it was of interest to compare the levels of superoxide dismutase in normal and schizophrenic brain.

Superoxide dismutase activity was measured in homogenates of control and schizophrenic diencephalon according to the method of McCord and Fridovich (1969). In rat brain, the level of the enzyme increased and then decreased during a 3-day postmortem period (figure 1). No difference in enzyme activity was found in age-matched groups of normal and schizophrenic subjects (table 5).

Choline acetyltransferase. Choline acetyltransferase catalyzes the synthesis of acetylcholine and brain levels of the enzyme may be used as a marker of central cholinergic activity (Fonnum, 1969). In human brain, choline acetyltransferase was found to have an unequal regional distribu-

Table 4

Monoamine oxidase activity in postmortem specimens of brain[a]

Group	Number of Cases	Mean Activity ± S.E.		
		Pons-Medulla	Diencephalon	Hippocampus
		Total Sample		
Control	12	1.75 ± 0.102	1.80 ± 0.081[b]	1.95 ± 0.096
Schizophrenic	18	1.99 ± 0.081	1.93 ± 0.089	1.98 ± 0.121
		Age Matched Sample		
Control	9	1.79 ± 0.132	1.79 ± 0.103	1.98 ± 0.100
Schizophrenic	14	1.98 ± 0.101	1.87 ± 0.099	1.98 ± 0.125

[a]Enzyme activity is expressed as μmol product per g tissue per hr. Assay of Wurtman and Axelrod, 1963. S.E., Standard error of mean.

[b]Number of cases = 11

Table 5

Superoxide dismutase activity in the diencephalon of schizophrenic patients and normal controls[a]

Group	Number of Cases	Mean Activity ± S.E.
Control	7	0.83 ± 0.038
Schizophrenic	8	0.88 ± 0.063

[a]Enzyme activity is expressed as arbitrary enzyme units (see McCord and Fridovich, 1969). S.E., standard error of mean.

tion; in contrast to DBH, choline acetyltransferase activity was lowest in the pons-medulla, intermediate in hippocampus, and highest in the diencephalon (table 6). A significant reduction in choline acetyltransferase activity was obtained in all 3 regions of schizophrenic brain, but the differences were in part due to the younger average age of the controls. Choline acetyltransferase activity varied inversely with age; the correlation between diencephalic enzyme level and age in the control group was -0.67. After matching the schizophrenic and control groups for age, a significant deficit was observed only in the hippocampus (table 6).

Catechol-O-methyl transferase. Catechol-O-methyl transferase (COMT) is a major enzyme in the metabolism of catecholamines and is thought to be "closely associated with adrenergic receptors" (Axelrod, 1968). If so, measurements of COMT in the brain could provide information about the postsynaptic component of central NE systems. Individual values of COMT in postmortem samples of human brain were highly replicable, but varied over a 10-fold range in both groups. Despite the large individual variation, there was a significant reduction in diencephalic COMT in the schizophrenic group (table 7); in the pons-medulla, the difference between the two groups was not statistically significant. In normal brain, COMT activity in the diencephalon significantly exceeded that in the pons-medulla ($P < .01$). This regional distribution is the reverse of that found for

Table 6

Choline acetyltransferase activity in the brains of schizophrenic patients and normal controls[a]

Group	Number of Cases	Mean Activity ± S.E.		
		Pons-Medulla	Diencephalon	Hippocampus
		Total Sample		
Control	12	0.18 ± 0.04	1.45 ± 0.22	0.38 ± 0.08
Schizophrenic	18	0.10 ± 0.02[b]	0.80 ± 0.11[c]	0.13 ± 0.02[c]
		Age Matched Sample		
Control	9	0.14 ± 0.04	1.08 ± 0.11	0.27 ± 0.05
Schizophrenic	14	0.09 ± 0.01	0.83 ± 0.12	0.13 ± 0.03[b]

[a]Enzyme activity is expressed as μmol product per g tissue per hr. Assay of Fonnum, 1969.
[b]Differs from control, P <05.
[c]P <.01.

Table 7

Catechol-O-methyl transferase activity in the brains of schizophrenic patients and normal controls[a]

Group	Mean Activity ± S.E.	
	Pons-Medulla (N)	Diencephalon (N)
Control	5.25 ± 0.73 (11)	7.42 ± 1.33 (11)
Schizophrenic	4.27 ± 0.87 (17)	4.31 ± 0.87 (18)[b]

[a]Enzyme activity is expressed as nmol product per g tissue per hr. Assay of Axelrod and Cohn, 1971. S.E., standard error of mean. N, number of cases.

[b]Differs from control, $P < .05$.

DBH, but it is consistent with the fact that NE terminals and receptors are concentrated in rostral regions of the brain. Interestingly, in the schizophrenic group, COMT activity in the diencephalon did not exceed that in the pons-medulla. Calculation of regional difference scores (diencephalon minus pons-medulla) for each subject confirmed the selective deficit of diencephalic COMT in the schizophrenic group. The differences between regions differed significantly in the two groups ($P < .01$).

Discussion

The results of our enzymatic studies may be summarized in order of importance as follows: 1) There was a significant reduction in the DBH activity of the schizophrenic group in all brain regions examined. The DBH deficits in hippocampus and diencephalon were somewhat larger than that in pons medulla. 2) There also were significant reductions of diencephalic COMT and hippocampal choline acetyltransferase activity in the schizophrenic group. However, individual values of COMT varied widely, and the activity of choline acetyltransferase was markedly dependent on age; hence, these deficits must be regarded as provisional until verified in larger samples. 3) There were no differences between the normal and schizophrenic groups in the activities of 3 enzymes: lactate dehydrogenase, monoamine oxidase and superoxide dismutase. These negative findings make it unlikely that gross artifacts were responsible for the enzymatic deficits that were observed.

The concept that schizophrenia may involve a deficit in DBH function is supported by the frequent observation of psychosis in alcoholics after overdoses of the DBH inhibitor, disulfiram. According to Angst (1956) disulfiram psychosis can be symptomatically indistinguishable from schizophrenia. Furthermore, Heath _et al_. (1965) report that disulfiram produces extreme mental and physical changes, including an increase in psychotic symptoms, in schizophrenic patients, but at comparable doses only minimal changes in prisoner control group.

The DBH deficits in the schizophrenic group may be explained in several ways. For example, it is possible that schizophrenics' DBH is different from and, hence, intrinsically less active than normal enzyme; however, similarities in the physiochemical properties and assay parameters of the 2 enzymes do not support this idea (Wise and Stein, 1973). It is also unlikely that the schizophrenics' DBH deficit was due to an excess of endogenous inhibitors. These would have been inactivated in the assay, and dialysis of homogenates did not affect the activity of the enzyme. The deficits could be the result of a defect in the synthesis or utilization of DBH, or they could reflect a more general pathological condition of NE neurons. As has already been suggested (Stein and Wise, 1971; Kety, 1972b), a defect in dopamine hydroxylation could lead to both an insufficiency of NE and an excess of dopamine at NE synapses. It is also possible that the NE neurons themselves are disturbed, or damaged, or fail to develop normally in schizophrenia. Furthermore, because regions rich in nerve terminals exhibited larger reductions in DBH than regions rich in cell bodies, it seems possible that the NE nerve terminal may be particularly susceptible to the schizophrenic disease process. Such vulnerability of terminals would be consistent with a suggestion that the schizophrenic process involves the formation of a toxic metabolite of dopamine, such as 6-hydroxydopamine (Stein and Wise, 1971) or dopamine _o_-quinone (Adams, 1972; Stein _et al_., 1972). As already noted, 6-hydroxydopamine has been shown in studies on animals to cause selective damage to central catecholamine nerve endings.

Interpretation of the choline acetyltransferase deficits must be even more speculative. However, a central cholinergic deficit in schizophrenia is consistent with a) biochemical evidence that cholinergic and noradrenergic neurons in sympathetic ganglia are developmentally and functionally interdependent (Black et al., 1971; Thoenen, 1972) and b) physiological evidence that autonomic disturbances in schizophrenia may involve both adrenergic and cholinergic dysfunction (Gruzelier and Venables, 1972; Rubin and Barry, 1972).

Needless to say, in view of the many false hopes and disappointments that biochemical studies of schizophrenia have produced, our findings must be viewed with skepticism until other researchers provide confirmation. A number of investigators have found normal levels of DBH in the blood serum of schizophrenics (Dunner et al., 1973; Lamprecht et al., 1973; Shopsin et al., 1972). However, catecholamine-related enzymes can be increased in the brain without concomitant peripheral changes (Lamprecht et al., 1972) and almost complete elimination of brain DBH by intraventricularly administered 6-hydroxydopamine had no effect on plasma DBH (Lamprecht et al., 1973). Hence, the level of DBH in plasma cannot be used as a measure of that in brain.

The single attempt to replicate the Wise and Stein (1973) observations produced ambiguous results. Wyatt et al. (1975) found small DBH deficits in the brains of schizophrenics that ranged from 11 to 23 percent, depending on the region examined. However, only the deficit in hippocampus approached statistical significance. Wyatt et al. also found a significant negative correlation between dose of medication and DBH activity in the schizophrenic group. Since recommended drug dosage depends in part on the severity of illness (Physicians' Desk Reference, 1974), this finding may indicate that a positive relationship exists between the severity of the illness and the deficit in DBH.

Although Wyatt et al. (1975) attribute their small deficits to postmortem factors and conclude that their data are "in discrepancy" with ours, we are inclined to believe that Wyatt's data and our own differ only in degree (Wise and Stein, 1975). To buttress the latter view, a plausible explanation should be provided for the disparity in the size of the deficits observed in the 2 studies. At least some forms of schizophrenia are chronic illnesses, which, in the pre-phenothiazine era, often progressed to profound deterioration (Bleuler, 1911). The biochemical approach to schizophrenia assumes that there are brain substrates which are the target of the disease process, and that the resulting disturbances in brain biochemistry are responsible for the behavioral pathology. If so, and if DBH-containing neurons were such a substrate, then the activity of the enzyme would decline as the disease progressed. Furthermore, if phenothiazine medication actually prevented or retarded the clinical deterioration (Klein and Davis, 1969), then the drugs, directly or indirectly, might also retard the neurochemical deterioration. The mean age at death of the schizophrenic patients in Wyatt's experiment was 49.2 years, compared to 71.2 years in our study; thus, assuming similarity of age at onset, the average duration of illness of our patients exceeded that of Wyatt's patients by 22 years. Furthermore, most of our patients had been ill for many years prior to 1952 when the phenothiazines were introduced; hence, our patients could have received no effective medication during the critical period of their illness. On the other hand, most of Wyatt's patients probably had received phenothiazines even at an early stage of illness. These considerations may account in part for the smaller DBH deficits exhibited by Wyatt's patients.

Finally, some therapeutic implications of our findings may be noted. The general aim would be to correct or compensate for the presumed pathology of NE systems. One could try to increase the formation of DBH, or to promote supersensitivity of NE receptors (Stein et al., 1972), or even, ideally, to stimulate the regeneration of damaged NE terminals as, for example, by suitable central administration of nerve growth factor (Björklund and Stenevi, 1972; Berger et al., 1973). Alternatively, in analogy to the use of L-DOPA to elevate the central levels of dopamine in Parkonsin's disease (Cotzias et al., 1967; Hornykiewicz, 1972), one could try to increase the concentration of NE in the brains of schizophrenic patients by administration of a precursor.[1]

Footnote

[1]Although high doses of L-DOPA have been found to exacerbate psychotic symptoms (Murphy, 1972), a beneficial effect in schizophrenic patients of moderate doses of L-DOPA in combination with phenothiazines has also been reported (Inanaga et al., 1972). It might be advantageous, however in view of the schizophrenic deficit in DBH, to bypass the dopamine step and to form NE directly from dihydroxyphenylserine, or from a related substance that will form NE more rapidly.

Acknowledgements

We thank J. Axelrod and R. Weinshilboum for guidance in setting up the DBH assay and M.M. Baden and M.H. Book for advice in selecting and obtaining human brain specimens. We also thank D.J. Reis for providing samples of phenylethanolamine-N-methyltransferase and A.T. Shropshire, W.J. Carmint, N.S. Buonato, and B.A. Tallardy for technical assistance.

References

Adams, R.N.: Stein and Wise theory of schizophrenia: A possible mechanism for 6-hydroxydopamine formation _in vivo_. Behav. Biol. 7: 861-866, 1972.

Angst, A.: Zur Frage der Psychosen bein Behandlung mit Disulfiram (Antabus). Schwiez. Med. Wochenschr. 46: 1304-1306, 1956.

Axelrod, J.: The fate of norepinephrine and the effect of drugs. The Physiologist 11: 63-73, 1968.

Axelrod, J.: Dopamine-β-hydroxylase: Regulation of its synthesis and release from nerve terminals. Pharmacol. Rev. 24: 233-243, 1972.

Axelrod, J. and Cohn, C.K.: Methyltransferase enzymes and red blood cells. J. Pharmacol. Exp. Ther. 176: 650-654, 1971.

Berger, B.D., Wise, C.D. and Stein, L.: Nerve growth factor: Enhanced recovery of feeding after hypothalamic damage. Science 180: 506-508, 1973.

Björklund, A. and Stenevi, U.: Nerve growth factor: Stimulation of regenerative growth of central noradrenergic neurons. Science 175: 1251-1252, 1972.

Black, I.B., Hendry, I. and Iversen, L.L.: Trans-synaptic regulation of growth and development of adrenergic neurones in mouse sympathetic ganglion. Brain Res. 34: 229-240, 1971.

Bleuler, E.: Dementia Praecox or the Group of Schizophrenias, 1911. Translated by J. Zinkin, International Universities Press, New York, 1950.

Bonnay, M., Troll, W. and Goldstein, M.: A radioassay for dopamine-β-hydroxylase (D-β-H) activity in tissues. Fed. Proc. 29: 278, 1970

Cotzias, G.C., Van Woert, M.H. and Schiffer, L.M.: Aromatic amino acids and modification of Parkinsonism. N. Engl. J. Med. 76: 374-379, 1967.

Dunner, D.L., Cohn, C.K., Weinshilboum, R.M. and Wyatt, R.J.: The activity of dopamine-beta-hydroxylase and methionine-activating enzyme in blood of schizophrenic patients. Biol. Psychiat. 6: 215-220, 1973.

Fonnum, F.: Radiochemical microassays for the determination of choline acetyltransferase and acetylcholinesterase activities. Biochem. J. 115: 465-472, 1969.

Fridovich, I.: Superoxide radical and superoxide dismutase. Acct. Chem. Res. 5: 321-326, 1972.

Fuxe, K., Goldstein, M., Hökfelt, M. and Joh, T.H.: Immunohistochemical localization of dopamine-β-hydroxylase in the peripheral and central nervous system. Res. Commun. Chem. Pathol. Pharmacol. 1: 627-636, 1970.

Gruzelier, J.H. and Venables, P.H.: Skin conductance orienting activity in a heterogenous sample of schizophrenics. J. Nerv. Ment. Dis. 155: 277-287, 1972.

Hartman, B.K. and Udenfriend, S.: The application of immunological techniques to the study of enzymes regulating catecholamine synthesis and degradation. Pharmacol. Rev. 24: 311-330, 1972.

Heath, R.G., Nesselhof, W., Bishop, M.P. and Byers, L.W.: Behavioral and metabolic changes associated with administration of tetraethylthiuram disulfide (Antabuse). Dis. Nerv. Syst. 26: 99-105, 1965.

Heikkila, R.E. and Cohen, G.: 6-Hydroxydopamine: Evidence for superoxide radical as an oxidative intermediate. Science 181: 456-457, 1973.

Hillarp, N.A., Fuxe, K. and Dahlström, A.: Demonstration and mapping of central neurons containing dopamine, noradrenaline, 5-hydroxytryptamine and their reactions to psychopharmaca. Pharmacol. Rev. 18: 727-741, 1966.

Hornykiewicz, O.: Dopamine and extrapyramidal motor function and dysfunction. In Neurotransmitters, ed. by I.J. Kopin, pp. 390-415, Williams and Wilkins, Baltimore, 1972.

Inanaga, K., Inoue, K., Tachibana, H., Oshima, M. and Kotorii, T.: Effects of L-DOPA in schizophrenia. Folia Psychiat. Neurol. Jap. 26: 145-158, 1972.

Johnson, M.K.: The intracellular distribution of glycolytic and other enzymes in rat-brain homogenates and mitochondrial preparations. Biochem. J. 77: 610, 1960.

Kaufman, S. and Friedman, S.: Dopamine-β-hydroxylase. Pharmacol. Rev. 17: 71-100, 1965.

Kety, S.S.: Brain catecholamines, affective states and memory. In The Chemistry of Mood, Motivation, and Memory, ed. by J.L. McGaugh, pp. 65-80, Plenum Press, New York, 1972a.

Kety, S.S.: Toward hypotheses for a biochemical component in the vulnerability to schizophrenia. Sem. Psychiat. 4: 233-238, 1972b.

Klein, D.F. and Davis, J.M.: Diagnosis and Drug Treatment of Psychiatric Disorders, pp. 139-161, Williams and Wilkins, Baltimore, 1969.

Kornberg, A.: Methods in Enzymology 1: 361, 1955.

Lamprecht, F., Eichelman, B., Thoa, N.B., Williams, R.B. and Kopin, I.J.: Rat fighting behavior: Serum dopamine-β-hydroxylase and hypothalamic tyrosine hydroxylase. Science 177: 1214-1215, 1972.

Lamprecht, F., Wyatt, R.J., Belmaker, R., Murphy, D.L. and Pollin, W.: Plasma dopamine-β-hydroxylase in identical twins discordant for schizophrenia. In Frontiers in Catecholamine Research, ed. by E. Usdin and S.H. Snyder, pp. 1123-1126, Pergamon Press, New York, 1973.

Lindvall, O. and Björklund, A.: The organization of the ascending catecholamine neuron systems in the rat brain as revealed by the glyoxylic acid fluorescence method. Acta Physiol. Scand., Supplement 412, 1-48, 1974.

McCord, J.M. and Fridovich, I.: Superoxide dismutase. J. Biol. Chem. 244: 6049-6055, 1969.

Miller, N.E.: Experiments on motivation. Science 126: 1271-1278, 1957.

Molinoff, P.B., Brimijoin, W.S., Weinshilboum, R.M. and Axelrod, J.: Neurally mediated increase in dopamine-β-hydroxylase activity. Proc. Nat. Acad. Sci. U.S.A. 66: 453-458, 1970.

Molinoff, P.B., Weinshilboum, R. and Axelrod, J.: A sensitive enzymatic assay for dopamine-β-hydroxylase. J. Pharmacol. Exp. Ther. 178: 425-431, 1971.

Murphy, D.L.: L-DOPA, behavioral activation and psychopathology. In Neurotransmitters, ed. by I.J. Kopin, p. 472, Williams and Wilkins, Baltimore, 1972.

Murphy, D.L. and Wyatt, R.J.: Reduced monoamine oxidase activity in blood platelets from schizophrenic patients. Nature 238: 225-226, 1972.

Neff, N.H., Yang, H.-Y.T., Goridis, C. and Bialek, D.: The metabolism of indolealkylamines by type A and B monoamine oxidase of brain. In Advances in Biochemical Psychopharmacology, Vol. 11, ed. by E. Costa, G.L. Gessa and M. Sandler, pp. 51-58, Raven Press, New York, 1974.

Olds, J.: Hypothalamic substrates of reward. Physiol. Rev. 42: 554-604, 1962.

Physician's Desk Reference, 28th Edition, p. 969, p. 1327, Medical Economics, Oradell, New Jersey, 1974.

Rado, S.: Psychoanalysis of Behavior, Vol. 2, Grune and Stratton, New York, 1962.

Reis, D.J. and Molinoff, P.B.: Brain dopamine-β-hydroxylase: Regional distribution and effects of lesions and 6-hydroxydopamine on activity. J. Neurochem. 19: 195-204, 1972.

Ritter, S. and Stein, L.: Self-stimulation in the mesencephalic trajectory of the ventral noradrenergic bundle Brain Res. 81: 145-157, 1974.

Ross, S.B., Weinshilboum, R., Molinoff, P.B., Vesell, E.S. and Axelrod, J.: Electrophoretic properties of dopamine-β-hydroxylase in several tissues from three species. Mol. Pharmacol. 8: 50-58, 1972.

Rubin, L.S. and Barry, T.J.: The reactivity of the iris muscles as an index of autonomic dysfunction in schizophrenic remission. J. Nerv. Ment. Dis. 155: 265-276, 1972.

Shopsin, B., Freedman, L.S., Goldstein, M. and Gershon, S.: Serum dopamine-β-hydroxylase (DβH) activity and affective states. Psychopharmacologia 27: 11-16, 1972.

Stein, L.: Self-stimulation of the brain and the central stimulant action of amphetamine. Fed. Proc. 23: 836-850, 1964.

Stein, L.: Chemistry of reward and punishment. In Psychopharmacology, A Review of Progress: 1957-1967, ed. by D.H. Efron, pp. 105-123, U.S. Government Printing Office, Washington, D.C., 1968.

Stein, L.: Norepinephrine reward pathways. Nebraska Symposium on Motivation 22: 113-129, 1975.

Stein, L. and Wise, C.D.: Possible etiology of schizophrenia: Progressive damage to the noradrenergic reward system by 6-hydroxydopamine. Science 171: 1032-1036, 1971.

Stein, L., Wise, C.D. and Berger, B.D.: Noradrenergic reward mechanisms, recovery of function, and schizophrenia. In The Chemistry of Mood, Motivation, and Memory, ed. by J.L. McGaugh, pp. 81-103, Plenum Publishing Corporation, New York, 1972.

Thoenen, H.: Comparison between the effect of neuronal activity and nerve growth factor on the enzymes involved in the synthesis of norepinephrine. Pharmacol. Rev. 24: 255-267, 1972.

Wise, C.D., Baden, M.M. and Stein, L.: Postmortem measurement of enzymes in human brain: Evidence of a central noradrenergic deficit in schizophrenia. J. Psychiat. Res. 11: 185-198, 1974.

Wise, C.D. and Stein, L.: Facilitation of brain self-stimulation by central administration of norepinephrine. Science 163: 299-301, 1969.

Wise, C.D. and Stein, L.: Dopamine-β-hydroxylase deficits in the brains of schizophrenic patients. Science 181: 344-347, 1973.

Wise, C.D. and Stein, L.: "Dopamine-β-hydroxylase activity in the brains of chronic schizophrenic patients", reply to Wyatt, Schwartz, Erdelyi and Barchas. Science 187: 370, 1975.

Wurtman, R.J. and Axelrod, J.: A sensitive and specific assay for the estimation of monoamine oxidase. Biochem. Pharmacol. 12: 1439-1441, 1963.

Wyatt, R.J., Murphy, D.L., Belmaker, R., Cohen, S., Donnelly, C.H. and Pollin, W.: Reduced monoamine oxidase activity in platelets: A possible genetic marker for vulnerability to schizophrenia. Science 179: 916-918, 1973.

Wyatt, R.J., Schwartz, M.A., Erdelyi, E. and Barchas, J.D.: Dopamine-β-hydroxylase activity in the brains of chronic schizophrenic patients. Science 187: 368-370, 1975.

Neurotransmitter Balances Regulating Behavior, edited and published by E.F. Domino and J.M. Davis, Ann Arbor, © 1975

NEUROTRANSMITTER BALANCES AND BEHAVIOR

Peter B. Dews
Laboratory of Psychobiology
Harvard Medical School
Boston, Massachusetts

The present discussion will add a new problem to the many concerned with the pharmacology of reward systems.

Back in the early days of psychopharmacology before ACNP was born, a procedure variously called conditioned suppression, conditioned emotional response (CER), Estes-Skinner paradigm and so on, became popular in drug studies. The original Estes-Skinner procedure (Estes and Skinner, 1941) had been to have rats working under a fixed-interval schedule (FI) for food, a procedure generating a steady state of responding on a lever (in those experiments), and then to superimpose an occasional, relatively short stimulus, concluding with an electric shock. The rats came to slow down and stop responding during the short stimulus. Estes and Skinner suggested the slow-down indicated "anxiety." Be that as it may, in the hands first of Brady and Hunt (1955) and then of many others, usually using a VI rather than an FI as background schedule, the procedure became a popular means of assessing drug effects and is generally familiar.

Sidman _et al_. (1957) asked the question: What will happen if the Estes-Skinner paradigm is superimposed on a steady rate of responding maintained not by VI food, but by a continuous shock avoidance schedule producing a similarly sustained steady responding? The results were clear cut. Instead of slowing down of responding during the stimulus preceding the unavoidable shock, there developed an increased rate of responding right up to the shock. There were plausible explanations of the phenomena that did not violate people's prejudices so the experiments were not denounced. The findings were confirmed by Kelleher _et al_. (1963), who went one step further. They eliminated the continuous avoidance component of the schedule. That is, for most of the session the squirrel monkeys were in a situation in which nothing happened, whether they did or did not press the lever; then a stimulus appeared for a short time concluded by a shock, again, whether or not the squirrel monkey pressed the lever. What happened was that the squirrel monkey stopped pressing the lever except when the stimulus was present; during the stimulus, the squirrel monkey continued to press right up to the shock

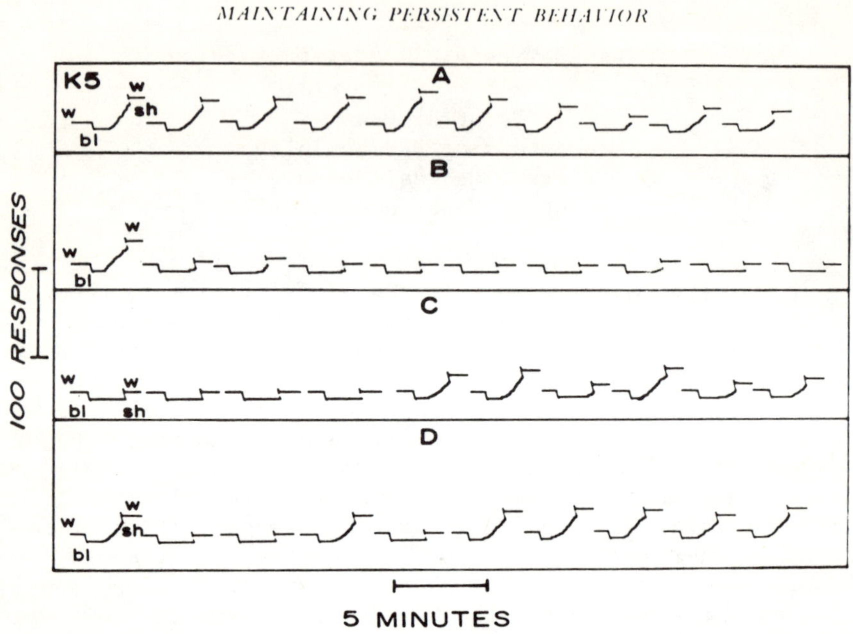

Fig. 1. Responding in a squirrel monkey under a schedule of unavoidable shock. Records show cumulated responding against time. A white light was present except when down-setting of recorder pen shows onset of a blue light which persisted for 2 min and terminated coincidental with an electric shock (rows A,C and D). In B the schedule was similar except no shocks were delivered. Note in A the progressive responding up to the shock and the relatively rapid disappearance of responding when the shock was discontinued in B, its reinstatement in the first session in which the shock was reintroduced (C) and the re-establishment after a number of sessions of the steady state pattern seen in A. (Reproduced by permission from Kelleher, R.T., Riddle, W.C. and Cook, L.: J. Exp. Anal. Behav. 6: 507-517, 1963. Copyright, 1963 by the Society for the Experimental Analysis of Behavior, Inc.)

(see figure 1). So Kelleher et al. demonstrated maintenance of responding simply by the presentation of unavoidable shocks. The behavior, however, was a little erratic from subject to subject, there was some doubt that it would continue indefinitely, so people were able to reconcile their prejudices with the findings by assuming the animals had been "tricked" into doing something "silly", and the experiments were not denounced.

In an independent sequence of experiments, Azrin was making systematic studies of punishment, punishment being defined as the presentation of a noxious stimulus when a response occurred. He (Azrin, 1960) showed that when an electric shock was presented every time a response occurred (responding being maintained by a VI schedule) there were graded reductions in the rate of responding, depending on the intensity of the shock. Kelleher and Morse (1968) were interested in developing patterns of responding which were the converse of FI responding. Under FI there is, to a first approximation, a progressive increase in rate of responding through the interval; the rate starts low at the beginning and reaches its maximum towards the end of the interval. Kelleher and Morse were interested in a pattern of responding in which the maximum rate was at the beginning of an interval and the rate then declined, reaching a minimum at the end of the interval. Since Azrin had shown how punishment could reduce responding, Kelleher and Morse decided to get their pattern of responding as follows (see figure 2). Responding was developed and maintained at a good rate in squirrel monkeys by a schedule for VI food. Then it was arranged that during each 11th min, every response would be followed by an electric shock to the tail of the subject. They thought that the suppressing effects of punishment might generalize backwards so that responding would decelerate as the 10 min period progressed to reach a minimum in the later part of the interval - the converse of the typical FI. They found that responding was effectively suppressed in the 11th min, when every response was shocked (Kelleher and Morse, 1968), just as Azrin's work had suggested it would. During the preceding 10 min, however, the rate of responding tended to increase and what is more, reached its highest levels just before the first response was shocked at the beginning of the 11th min, just the opposite of what they had been looking to get. Steady responding occurred at a rate appropriate to get the food VI for the first few minutes of the 10 min period, and then there was a change, in most periods, to a considerably higher rate which was then maintained until a shock was delivered; there were then very few responses in the 11th min. In most of the experiments, everything was turned off during the 12th min, and then the whole cycle repeated with the same pattern of behavior repeating. Kelleher and Morse took the next step: they eliminated the food schedule (see figure 3). The result was that responding more or less ceased at the beginning of the interval, then accelerated and the maximum rate occurred in the last part of the interval as the time for shock

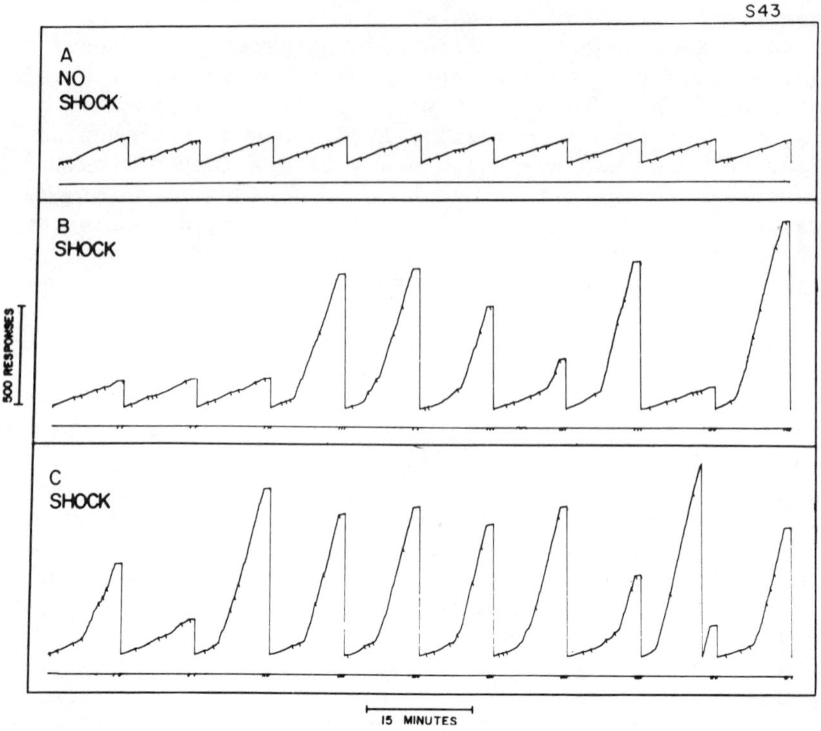

Fig. 2. Effects of scheduled electric shock on responding of squirrel monkey. Abscissa: time. Ordinate: cumulative responding, resetting every 660 sec. A. Responding under a schedule of irregular intermittent reinforcement of responses by delivery of food (VI 120 sec). Note the steady rate of responding throughout session. Food deliveries shown by hatch marks on record. B and C. The first two consecutive sessions after a shock schedule was reintroduced, superimposed on food schedule. The schedule was delivery of a shock of 12.6 ma to the tail of the monkey at the first response after 600 sec and then at every response during the next 60 sec. Notice that after only 3 shock deliveries, at start of B, there is large increase in rate of responding over that under the food schedule alone, positively accelerated up to the shock, showing the positive reinforcing properties of the shock. Thereafter, for the next 60 sec, there are very few responses, many fewer than under the food schedule alone, showing that the same shock as that showing positive reinforcing properties, can, under a different schedule, suppress responding. (Reproduced by permission from Kelleher, R.T. and Morse, W.H.: J. Anal. Behav. 11: 819-838, 1968, modified Fig. 4. Copyright, 1968 by the Society for the Experimental Analysis of Behavior, Inc.)

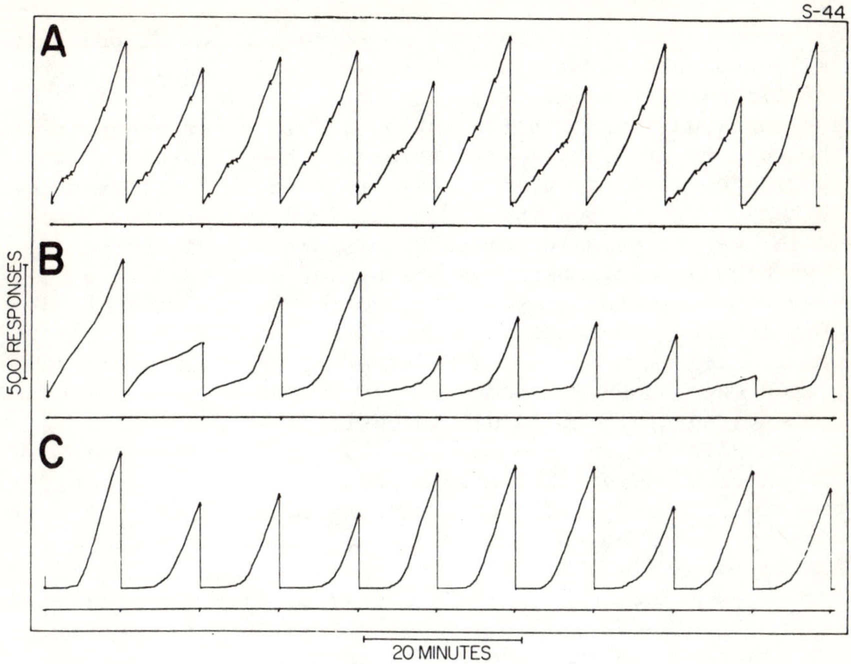

Fig. 3. Development of FI pattern of responding with electric shock as reinforcer. Abscissa: time. Ordinate: cumulative responding, resetting every 600 sec. A. Concurrent food and shock schedule. Irregular food deliveries shown by hatch marks on record (VI 120 sec), shock delivered every 600 sec at a response whereupon pen reset. Notice that responding continued throughout session but that the rate increased as the time of shock approached. B. Next session. Food schedule discontinued, so only consequence of responding is delivery of shock every 600 sec. Decline of rate of responding early in the interval is apparently already in the 3rd and 4th intervals, showing extinction of the food maintained responding, leaving the shock as the sole positive reinforcer. C. Sixty sessions later. During each of the intervening sessions the subject delivered 10 shocks at 600 sec intervals, the shock being the only consequence of the responding. The result of the total of the 100 hr of exposure to the schedule is a smoothly accelerating, highly characteristic pattern of FI responding, indistinguishable from that seen with food or other conventional positive reinforcers. (Reproduced by permission from Kelleher, R.T. and Morse, W.H.: J. Exp. Anal. Behav. 11: 819-838, 1969, from Figs. 18 and 19. Copyright, 1969 by the Society for the Experimental Analysis of Behavior, Inc.)

delivery approached; that is, an FI pattern developed just as though food rather than shock were being delivered at the first response after the end of a 10 min FI period. The shock was thus functioning as a reinforcer since it was the only event maintaining responding and it produced a pattern of responding like that produced by familiar reinforcers. The responding was maintained indefinitely. One monkey was exposed to some 170 sessions over a period approaching a year, making an average of over 4000 responses/session or a total of some 700,000 responses, maintained only by 1900 shocks of 12.6 ma. Shock-producing responding was reduced when shock was reduced in intensity and disappeared when shock was removed only to return when shock was re-instated at the original intensity.

Two points deserve emphasis. One is that these monkeys had never pressed a lever to avoid a shock. It is not, therefore, possible to attribute the maintenance of responding by shocks to spurious avoidance since there was no history of avoidance. Transfer of control of a response from food maintained to shock avoidance does not occur spontaneously. Second, in the later phases of the experiments the monkeys were fully fed, so that responding could not have been maintained by food deprivation.

The findings have been confirmed several times. Kelleher and Morse have developed shock maintained responding using entirely different schedules to engender the initial responding, so there is no concealed trick in the procedure itself (Kelleher and Morse, 1969). They have even developed shock-maintained responding without _any_ training by taking a response that tends to occur after delivery of a shock (pulling a leash) and making that produce a shock. When the production of shocks was put on an FI schedule, then FI patterns of leash-pulling developed (Morse _et al._, 1967). McKearney (1970) has shown that FR as well as FI can be maintained by response-produced shock and Byrd (1969) has shown the phenomenon in cats. In retrospect, one can find other instances in the literature of paradoxical effects of punishment, in which "punishment" increased responding. Because these experiments effectively contradict strongly held prejudices of determinants of behavior, they have been denounced and many have accepted absurdly contrived anthropomorphic "explanations" to avoid facing the implications.

What has all this got to do with the pharmacology of reward systems? In the search for the neurological substratum of reinforcement, there seems to be an implicit assumption of a hard-wired system. Certain types of stimuli, positively reinforcing stimuli, feed into a positively reinforcing system anatomically related to brain placements which lead to intracranial self-stimulation. Other types of stimuli feed into other places which maintain avoidance behavior or punishment effects. What maintenance of behavior by response-produced shocks shows is that positive or negative reinforcing properties cannot be assigned to stimuli in a unique way. Whether a given stimulus will function as a reinforcer or as a punisher depends on more than just the nature of the stimulus. Food and shock are very different sorts of stimuli. They have very different behavior properties. No suggestion is made that food and shock can be used interchangeably in general. Yet with specific reference to reinforcing function, they can, under certain circumstances, be interchangeable. They have very different pathways in the CNS. What is it about a stimulus that makes it able to reinforce? The answer is probably nothing about the stimulus itself except that it is distinctive and to some extent pre-emptive. A reasonable hypothesis seems to be that reinforcement has mostly to do with temporal relations between a response and a stimulus; stimuli at the right time after a response reinforce that response. After a response occurs there must be some sort of persisting trace of the activity in areas of the CNS which preceded, and determined, the discharge down motor nerves that produced the sequence of contractions of skeletal muscles that constituted the response. Presumably the trace is diffuse though perhaps mostly associated with neurones on the motor side of the CNS. Places in the brain that lead to intracranial self-stimulation would then become merely places where electric shocks can initiate excitation that reinforces, just as electric shocks to the monkey's periphery initiate excitation that reinforces. What evidence is there that stimuli delivered to self-stimulating places in the brain function in a qualitatively different way from stimuli delivered elsewhere? Studies have tended to emphasize their similarity. Self-stimulation phenomena are still well worth studying, but it should not be assumed that study of the pharmacology of ICSS is in some way study of something closer to the essence of the pharmacology of reward than is study of the behavioral pharmacology of schedule-controlled behavior with no electrodes in the brain.

Reward systems or reinforcement systems are systems whereby responses that are followed by appropriate consequences are made more likely to occur in the future. That such "systems" exist is indubitable, just as is biological evolution, but also, just like evolution <u>how</u> they operate is not obvious. It was earlier suggested that time relations may be fundamental. This, like Darwin's "survival of the fittest", is a statement of a determining relationship, not of mechanism (Darwinism had to wait for genetics to get insight into mechanism). Nevertheless, pinpointing the determining relationship may be a prerequisite for investigating mechanism.

Why time relations? In evolution, insects, for example, have become highly preprogrammed, hard-wired; that is, a given set of circumstances control a given behavior in the insect, with almost no regard for past experience. In primates, on the other hand, past experience is dominant in determining response in most situations. Look at a human driving a car. Almost everything is determined by experience, nothing inborn. Neither the stimuli that control - arbitrary red lights and arbitrary rules about not hitting people - nor the motor responses - infinitesimal movements of the right foot and reciprocal movements of the two hands - have any predriving plausibility. The primate, especially man, comes into the world with some behavioral activities and the potentiality for vastly more. How are these sorted out, some preferentially strengthened, others weakened, to fit the individual to function in a particular niche in nature and society, a niche which is different for every individual? We say by preferential reinforcement. It is things that do things, have consequence, that are reinforced. How do we know when some behavioral activity has done something to the environment? Why, because the consequences follow the response; it is a time relationship. Do A and it is followed (perhaps only sometimes) by B. B reinforces A. Now suppose the process of reinforcement operates faster than discrimination. That is not unreasonable. Discrimination involves comparisons with previous stimuli, so it presumably involves retrieval and comparison, activities which may well be slow. When the monkey shocks its tail, the brief shock (45 msec) occurs within msec of the completion of the response. The shock signals something important has happened and the trace of the response is reinforced. Subsequently, the monkey screams and thrashes around. The noxious nature of the stimulus is discriminated for what it is. But alas! It is too late. The response was reinforced in the first second (taking into account conduction times) and what happens subsequently is irrelevant.

These speculations should not be taken seriously until they are supported (or refuted) by evidence. They have one purpose here. To show that natural explanations of the maladaptive behavior of self-shocking are conceivable. But experiments on self-shock have got to be taken into account by anyone seeking explanations and mechanisms of systems of reward.

References

Azrin, N.H.: Effects of punishment intensity during variable-interval reinforcement. J. Exp. Anal. Behav. 3: 123-142, 1960.

Brady, J.V. and Hunt, H.F.: An experimental approach to the analysis of emotional behavior. J. Psychol. 40: 313-324, 1955.

Byrd, L.D.: Responding in the cat maintained under response independent electric shock and response-produced electric shock. J. Exp. Anal. Behav. 12: 1-10, 1969.

Estes, W.K. and Skinner, B.F.: Some quantitative properties of anxiety. J. Exp. Psychol. 29: 390-400, 1941.

Kelleher, R.T., Riddle, W.C. and Cook, L.: Persistent behavior maintained by unavoidance shocks. J. Exp. Anal. Behav. 6: 507-517, 1963.

Kelleher, R.T. and Morse, W.H.: Schedules using noxious stimuli. III. Responding maintained with response-produced electric shocks. J. Exp. Anal. Behav. 11: 819-838, 1968.

Kelleher, R.T. and Morse, W.H.: Schedules using noxious stimuli. IV. An interlocking shock-postponement schedule in the squirrel monkey. J. Exp. Anal. Behav. 12: 1063-1079, 1969.

McKearney, J.W.: Responding under fixed-ratio and multiple fixed-interval fixed-ratio schedules of electric shock presentation. J. Exp. Anal. Behav. 14: 1-6, 1970.

Morse, W.H., Mead, R.N. and Kelleher, R.T.: Modulation of elicited behavior by a fixed-interval schedule of electric shock presentation. Science 157: 215-217, 1967.

Sidman, M., Herrnstein, R.J. and Conrad, D.G.: Maintenance of avoidance behavior by unavoidable shocks. J. Comp. Physiol. Psychol. 50: 553-557, 1957.

Neurotransmitter Balances Regulating Behavior,
edited and published by E.F. Domino and
J.M. Davis, Ann Arbor, © 1975

CHOLINERGIC AND ADRENERGIC BALANCE IN MANIA AND SCHIZOPHRENIA

John M. Davis
Illinois State Psychiatric Institute
Chicago, Illinois
and Department of Psychiatry
University of Chicago
Chicago, Illinois

David Janowsky
University of California
School of Medicine at San Diego
La Jolla, California

Current biological models of mania, depression and schizophrenia have hypothesized that the cause of these disorders is a deficit in, or excess of, a single neurotransmitter. We might call these the single transmitter disease theories. While much of the evidence suggests that abnormalities in individual transmitters play a causal role in the development of these mental disorders, there are important arguments for considering the development of causal models that involve more than one transmitter or amine. It has been long recognized that elaborate homeostatic systems in organisms, involving intricate balances of various mutually regulating biochemical systems, control virtually every biologic function. In the case of mental disease, the functioning of the parasympathetic and the peripheral sympathetic nervous systems are particularly important. A balance between these two systems regulates peripheral autonomic functions. Furthermore, balances between different transmitters are implicated in the central hypothalamic control of the pituitary releasing factors.

Dopaminergic and Cholinergic Systems in Parkinson's Disease

The factors governing parkinsonian symptoms may provide an illustrative model of how several factors may combine to produce a psychiatric disorder. Parkinsonian symptoms have been associated with the depletion of dopamine in particular brain centers. Low dopamine levels in certain brain centers, for example, have been found in postmortem examinations of patients with Parkinson's disease. Pseudoparkinsonian symptoms are caused in normal persons by neuroleptic drugs which blockade the dopamine receptors. L-DOPA, which is converted to dopamine and raises the overall levels of this transmitter, has the opposite effect of reducing parkinsonian symptoms. Such findings suggest that dopamine is the principal causal factor in this disorder.

It is important to note, however, that a balance between the dopaminergic and the cholinergic systems influences parkinsonian symptoms. Therapeutic use is made of anticholinergic medication to reduce parkinsonian symptoms. Alternatively, physostigmine, which acts upon the cholinergic system by preventing the breakdown of acetylcholine and, hence, increases its brain levels, can intensify the symptoms of parkinsonian patients. However, according to our studies, physostigmine does not cause parkinsonian symptoms in normal patients. Consequently, it appears that the cholinergic system exercises a secondary modulating effect on this disorder. Thus, while the cholinergic system plays a modulating though not a causal role in the disorder, an adequate analysis of parkinsonian dysfunction must take into account the functional influences of the cholinergic as well as the adrenergic systems.

It is also important to emphasize that a balance of transmitters model may prove to be an important explanatory tool in our conceptualization of mental disease. Because balances of transmitters are implicated in so many physiologic functions, it is reasonable to inquire whether mania, depression, and schizophrenia may also involve an imbalance of transmitters.

Physostigmine and a Two Factor Theory of Depression and Mania

The catecholamine models of depression and mania are traditional, single transmitter theories which propose that depression is associated with low brain levels of norepinephrine and mania with abnormally high norepinephrine levels. Janowsky and I (Janowsky *et al.*, 1972), following the analogy with Parkinson's disease, hypothesized that the cholinergic system might be expected to modulate the primary effects of abnormalities in the noradrenergic system. The two factor hypothesis would then propose that depression would be associated with a low level of norepinephrine modulated by a high acetylcholine level. Mania would be associated with a high norepinephrine - low acetylcholine level (or function).

We reasoned that with manic patients we could bring about a reduction in mania by administering physostigmine, which produces increased brain levels of acetylcholine.

This procedure would produce changes (increased activity) in the cholinergic system to modulate the manic effects of an overactive noradrenergic system. We further hypothesized that physostigmine might also produce depression in patients with pre-existing affective disease.

Our subject population, selected after obtaining informed consent, consisted of both depressed and manic patients with schizophrenic patients as controls. Neostigmine was used as an active placebo in these studies to insure the integrity of the double blind design. Although it does not pass the blood-brain barrier, neostigmine, in proper doses, produces peripheral effects equivalent to those of physostigmine. Methylscopolamine was administered to protect patients against peripheral cholinergic toxicity.

Quantification of the degree of mania was obtained with the Beigel-Murphy Manic Rating Scale. Raters were blind as to whether patients received physostigmine or neostigmine. The course of effects of physostigmine over time are displayed in figure 1. This time course is consistent with the biologic half-life of physostigmine and its effects on brain acetylcholine in animals.

Administration of physostigmine in manic patients resulted in a dramatic reduction of the mania, whereas the placebo, neostigmine, produced no changes in the disorder (Janowsky et al., 1973c). With physostigmine, the mania was essentially converted to a psychomotor retarded depression. Initially, patients exhibited typical manic symptoms, i.e., rapidity of thought and movement, grandiose ideation, punning and rhyming, etc. Patients appeared lethargic following physostigmine and were significantly slower in their movement and speech. Patients reported subjective feelings of feeling drained and without energy, apathetic, and having "no thoughts in their head." Less consistently, the patient response to physostigmine was the feeling of depression. Some manic patients reported that they felt depressed following the drug while observers noted that a number cried and manifested other signs of depressed affect. Greater psychomotor retardation tended to characterize the more depressed patients.

Physostigmine had its most pronounced effect on the level of motoric activity and the rate of motor behavior. Mood was affected less consistently, with depressed affect occurring in some but not all patients. Some depressed affect, following medication with physostigmine or experimental cholinesterase inhibitors, occurred in patients in a normal volunteer study. A much greater degree of depressed affect following physostigmine occurred in patients with pre-existing affective disturbances than in schizophrenics

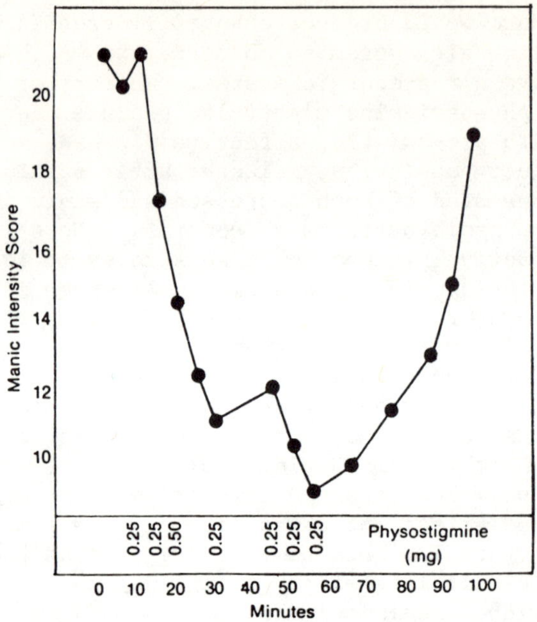

Fig. 1. Changes over time in Beigel-Murphy Manic Intensity Scale score for patients receiving 2 mg of physostigmine.

with no affect disorder. The finding suggests that there may be some specificity of physostigmine action (table 1).

It is clear, however, that a greater disturbance in rate than in affect or thought content is produced by physostigmine in acute doses. An explanation as to why the rate disturbance is altered to a greater degree than the mood and thought disturbance might take at least two forms. One explanation concerns the limited length of time during which physostigmine is active. Physostigmine effects are acute in nature, typically lasting about one hour. In spite of its effects on the other symptoms of mania, the very rapid nature of the physostigmine effect may, in part, be responsible for its failure to alter thought disorder. It may be that the nature of thought disorder is such that it would not be expected to undergo rapid alteration. For example, the highly agitated behavior of certain schizophrenic patients may often be reduced in a few hours by acute administration of phenothiazines, but the attendant thought disorder may take several weeks or months to ameliorate.

A second possible explanation might postulate pharmacol-

Table 1

Changes in symptom with physostigmine

Affective State	Control	Physostigmine	T	P
Beigel-Murphy Manic Intensity	15.30 ± 2.09	8.71 ± 1.24	3.67	<.002
Beigel-Murphy Euphoria	2.54 ± 0.49	0.73 ± 0.30	4.17	<.001
Talkative	2.98 ± 0.28	1.56 ± 0.19	4.16	<.001
Is Active	1.89 ± 0.30	0.83 ± 0.16	4.18	<.001
Cheerfulness	1.44 ± 0.19	0.45 ± 0.15	4.42	<.0007
Friendly	1.79 ± 0.17	1.10 ± 0.23	2.46	<.02
Grandiosity	0.38 ± 0.22	0.17 ± 0.11	1.16	NS
Flight of Ideas	1.98 ± 0.38	0.93 ± 0.24	3.62	<.0025
Happy	1.71 ± 0.26	0.38 ± 0.16	4.55	<.0006
Depressed	0.66 ± 0.20	1.68 ± 0.41	4.03	<.002

ogical distinctions between the several mental functions contributing to the same syndrome. Rate functions may be regulated by the amine-cholinergic balance to a greater extent than either the mood or thought functions. In other words, mania and depression may be disorders which involve more than one mental function and more than one transmitter. Hence, the cholinergic system may be implicated primarily in the rate disturbance while other systems are involved in other features of the disorder.

Necessarily, any discussion of the specificity of physostigmine action in manic-depressive disease is of a speculative nature. The cause of manic-depressive disease remains to be determined, as does the determination of which of its symptoms are the primary ones as opposed to the secondary. To the extent that the rate disturbances (being speeded up or slowed down) are considered primary in mania and depression, one would conclude that physostigmine is a relatively specific medication. If the core symptom of mania is posited to be the disturbance of thought content (such as having grandiose delusions), then physostigmine would be considered less specific. In our view, an assessment of physostigmine's specificity of action depends on assumptions about what is important in mania and depression. Those who put more emphasis on the rate disturbance in depression and mania are more impressed with its effects than those who consider the ideational components of mania and depression to be the essence of the disorder.

Nevertheless, it is important to note that physostigmine has antimanic effects which appear qualitatively different from those of sedation. Patients can remain manic while under heavy sedation. This development is frequently seen when clinically severe life threatening outbursts of manic excitement are treated with high doses of chlorpromazine or i.v. barbiturates. Highly sedating doses can leave patients obtunded and almost semicomatose. When they begin to emerge from the semicoma state, it is apparent that they remain acutely manic in all respects, in spite of their sedation. Markedly manic thinking and actions persist simultaneously with slurred speech, a staggering, toxic gait and other signs of heavy sedation. Physostigmine, on the other hand, has a direct effect on the mania without producing sedation. It would be inaccurate to propose that its action is that of nonspecific sedation as with the barbiturates.

Findings concerning the effects of physostigmine on mental functioning suggest the involvement of cholinergic systems in mania and depression. Further evidence of this involvement is to be found in the treatment domain. It is important to note that reserpine, for example, which can cause depression in hypertensive patients, has central cholinomimetic properties. The tricyclic antidepressants, the most effective category of antidepressants, have central anticholinergic properties. The anticholinergic properties of the tricyclic drugs may well be a helpful property and contribute to the therapeutic action in a secondary way. This interpretation seems particularly likely since attempts to develop "pure" antidepressants, which inhibit only the norepinephrine membrane pump without producing anticholinergic blockade, have been unsuccessful. Consequently, anticholinergic properties may exercise a therapeutic action in the treatment of depression. Hence, the concept that a single amine, norepinephrine, is the cause of depression may be incomplete with respect to what we know about how this disorder responds to medical treatment.

A Two Factor Model of Schizophrenia

Central to current biological theories of schizophrenia is the so-called dopamine theory, which implicitly suggests that abnormally high dopamine functions or levels are the primary causal factor in this disorder. The dopamine hypothesis is the single transmitter, single disease model of the etiology of schizophrenia.

Evidence supporting the dopamine theory of schizophrenia comes from two sources, one specific and one general. Specifically, all antipsychotic compounds block dopamine receptors. Generally, it is known that the antipsychotic action of all neuroleptics involves catecholamines, since *alpha*-methyl-*para*-tyrosine, a catecholamine synthesis inhibitor, potentiates the antipsychotic action of the neuroleptics.

Clinically, it has been noted that injections of psychomotor stimulants can intensify schizophrenia episodes, or even precipitate them in patients manifesting a latent schizophrenic disorder. For example, in double-blind studies of patients with active schizophrenic disorders, David Janowsky and I (Davis and Janowsky, 1973; Janowsky *et al.*, 1973a) compared the effects of placebo to small amounts of i.v. methylphenidate. The result produced by the methylphenidate was a marked worsening of the illness. Such a result also occurs with the administration of *d*- or *l*-amphetamine. The quantitative ratings of the severity of the psychosis were approximately doubled.

This intensification of psychosis with methylphenidate has been shown to be under the control of a dopaminergic-cholinergic balance. For example, physostigmine administered prior to methylphenidate prevents the further development of a methylphenidate-induced psychosis. Administered after the injection of methylphenidate, physostigmine terminates further intensification of the induced psychosis (though not of the underlying disorder). Figure 2 illustrates this (Janowsky et al., 1973b). However, what is of particular theoretical interest here is that similar doses of methylphenidate, when administered to normals, merely produce a mild euphoria. It appears that schizophrenic individuals are unusually sensitive to methylphenidate.

There are problems with a single transmitter theory of schizophrenia, however, since it leaves numerous factors unaccounted for. For this reason, and for heuristic purposes, I would like to formulate here an alternative to the single transmitter, single disease theory which proposes that schizophrenia is a consequence of excessive functional dopamine. This alternate formulation is a two factor theory of schizophrenia. One factor would involve some other cause, such as the CPK abnormality outlined in the work of Meltzer (Meltzer et al., 1970; Meltzer, 1974). The second factor would involve the dopaminergic system or, more probably, a dopaminergic-cholinergic balance. This factor would act by modulating the disturbance caused by the central factor in much the same way that the cholinergic system may modulate the movement disorder of Parkinson's disease and the rate disturbance of mania and depression. Thus, our two factors would consist of a central, and as yet unknown, factor and a second modulating factor under adrenergic-cholinergic control. If this is so, then antipsychotic agents, in blocking the dopamine receptors, re-establish a proper adrenergic-cholinergic balance and thereby inhibit the schizophrenic process. Such a reduction in the intensity of the schizophrenic symptoms may then permit the body's normal reparative mechanisms to work on other features of the disorder. In this way, the illness may remit over a period of several weeks as healing, in the broadest sense, takes place in the other pertinent systems.

At the present time, in the absence of more definitive evidence, the most substantial argument in support of a two factor theory concerns the course of time during which the neuroleptic drugs exercise their therapeutic benefits. This time course is illustrated in figure 3, which Dr. Cole and I prepared, based upon data from NIMH Collaborative Study No. 1. As can be seen from inspection of figure 3, the time course for recovery is rather long, indicating a slow recovery. I believe that this evidence is strongly suggestive of the operation of factors other than abnormalities in the dopaminergic-adrenergic system.

There are other clues which may be important in our modulation factor hypothesis. For example, certain

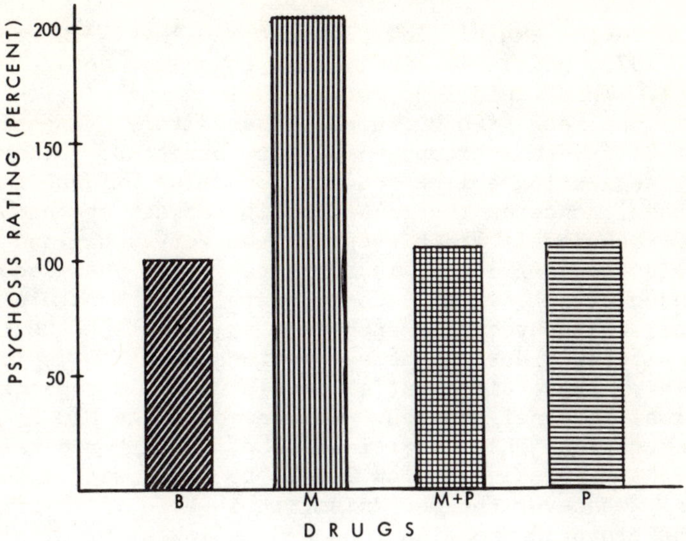

Fig. 2. Effects of methylphenidate (M), physostigmine (P), and methylphenidate and physostigmine (M + P) on psychosis rating (percent), as compared with baseline rating of 100 percent.

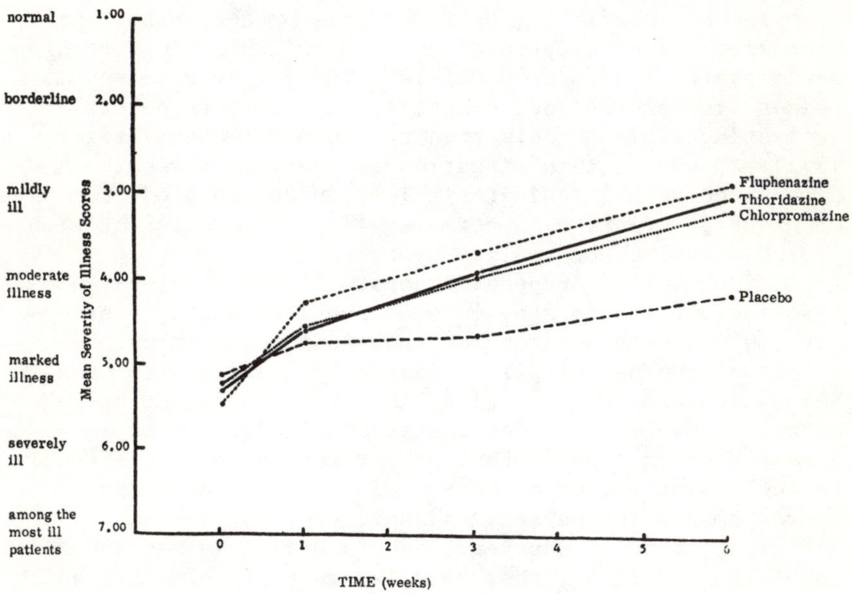

Fig. 3. Severity of illness over time in patients treated with phenothiazines. (Data from NIMH-PSC Collaborative Study I).

schizophrenics exhibit low platelet MAO levels (Murphy and Wyatt, 1972) and it is likely that this is under genetic control. This would lead to the obvious speculation that here is the mechanism by which an hereditary, dispositional vulnerability to schizophrenia is transmitted. Other evidence, suggesting a link between monoamine oxidase and schizophrenia, concerns the relationship between age and MAO level. MAO levels are highest in the very young and the very old, and are lowest in adolescents and young adults (Robinson et al., 1971). Coincidentally, the natural history of schizophrenia is such that it has its highest incidence precisely during the age periods when MAO is lowest. Certainly, these differential levels may be a consequence of normal hormonal changes. Furthermore, the MAO factor may be critical only in patients who, on an hereditary basis, have chronically low levels to begin with. Nevertheless, whatever the mechanism, it is both interesting and thought provoking to find that MAO is lowest precisely during the age period in which the incidence of schizophrenia is highest. This is consistent with my speculation that MAO may play a role in "factor 2" (the central, causal factor). Certainly, MAO as an intracellular enzyme is important in the regulation of intracellular amine levels.

There is additional data which implicates abnormalities in amine storage in the schizophrenia process. Both amphetamine and methylphenidate are excellent releasers of newly synthesized stored amines. The latter releases more amines from stores and, concomitantly, is more potent in activating schizophrenia than the former (Scheel-Krüger, 1971). However, this situation is specific to schizophrenics since methylphenidate is less potent in producing psychomotor stimulation in normals. This is consistent with a stored dopamine abnormality hypothesis.

A final bit of supportive data: Alpha-methyl-para-tyrosine blocks the synthesis of dopamine and is ineffective in treating schizophrenia, yet it potentiates the effect of the neuroleptics. Reserpine, which also posses-ses antipsychotic properties, interferes with the storage of dopamine. Thus, reserpine is most effective on amine stores whereas alpha-methyl-para-tyrosine is most effective on newly synthesized amines. This further implicates stored amines in the schizophrenic process.

Irrespective of whether these theories ultimately prove to be true or false, they have generated information which is important in clinical practice, since the pharmacologic concepts which underly these theories are useful in understanding drug side effects. For example, the concept of cholinergic blockade is useful in explaining the central anticholinergic syndrome. This syndrome can result when multiple anticholinergic agents are administered to psychiatric patients, resulting in an additive effect (El-Yousef et al., 1973).

In this paper, it has been suggested that there may be two or more factors which contribute to produce manic depressive illness or schizophrenia. In depression, cholinergic factors may modulate the hypothesized norepinephrine deficit. In schizophrenia, dopamine (or a dopaminergic-cholinergic balance) might serve to modulate a second, presently unknown factor, rather than playing a central role, as suggested by the dopamine theory. The blockade of dopamine by neuroleptics thus permits a normal reparative process to take place in connection with the second factor. It remains for us to discern what the central factor is. Considering manic depressive illness and schizophrenia to be the result of a two factor or multifactor process should emphasize their importance in distinguishing between those agents which might be the principal cause of a disorder and those secondary factors which serve to modulate the disorder.

Methodological Cautions

Several methodological cautions are appropriate at this point. First, although our reasoning is based upon pharmacologic evidence, its speculative and inferential nature should be apparent, and the theory should be regarded as such. Certainly, it is in no sense a well formed, systematically substantiated theory. It is important to label speculation as such because frequently by the time such speculative theory reaches the practitioner, it is taken to be established fact. It is appropriate to generate such theories for their heuristic value, but only if they are clearly labelled as speculative or, to borrow an apt phrase from Dr. Daniel X. Freedman, as "meta-neuropsychopharmacology."

The second methodological caution concerns the hypothesized low brain MAO level of schizophrenics. Many pharmacologic effects do not appear until MAO is almost completely inhibited. Hence, although lowering MAO to 1% of normal would be physiologically significant, there is reason to question whether lowering MAO by about 50 to 80% of normal is physiologically significant. This is an important criticism of the significance of low MAO levels in schizophrenia. Nevertheless, it is still possible that low platelet MAO is a clue to the biochemistry of schizophrenia, since patients possessing low platelet MAO might also manifest low central MAO to a degree that was physiologically significant. While this is unlikely, it is nevertheless possible. The fact that MAO is not completely inhibited does not mean that low MAO levels in schizophrenia are merely coincidental and irrelevant to the process of the disorder.

A third caution also relates to brain MAO levels. It has been noted earlier that there exists a curvilinear relationship between brain MAO level and age, with the highest levels occurring in young and old and the lowest levels occurring in adolescents and young adults. However, brain MAO levels obtained from postmortems of elderly schizophrenics are not necessarily an accurate representation of what these patients' MAO levels were when they were young and their illness was active. Thus, biochemical studies of brain amine levels, based upon an elderly, chronic psychiatric population, may not provide the basis for a good model of schizophrenia.

Finally, a fourth caution which applies equally to the biochemical theories of depression and schizophrenia, is that too frequently these theories are spoken of in terms of "turnover" or "level." The evidence which supports these theories is based, almost entirely, on pharmacologic studies. These studies do not point specifically to any particular mechanism. It is quite possible to suggest an alternative mechanism, that the causal mechanism is an impairment in the function of the norepinephrine receptor, rather than a low norepinephrine level or turnover which has been postulated to occur in depression. One must recognize that in speaking of low NE in depression or high DA in schizophrenia, one is really referring to dopaminergic or noradrenergic "function." Even qualifying one's terminology by referring to "free" norepinephrine in the synaptic cleft is not strictly supportable, since most of the evidence would be equally compatible with a theory that suggested that the defect was post-synaptic. Many defects could result in low noradrenergic function: (1) low amine levels, (2) low rates of amine synthesis, (3) defects at the receptor site, (4) defects in the amine release process, (5) alterations in membrane permeability and transport, and (6) excessive degradation or metabolic alterations which result in lower noradrenergic function (*e.g.*, excessive intracellular metabolism).

To summarize, we suggest that there may be alternative theories to the single transmitter, single disease models which are salient in present biological psychiatry. Most physiologic functions achieve homeostasis through a balance between neurophysiologic systems. The sympathetic-parasympathetic peripheral autonomic system is an excellent example. Likewise, systemic balance or imbalance may well play a central role in mental disorder. We have formulated an hypothesis and presented supportive empirical evidence that the central cholinergic system may well play a role in manic-depressive illness by modulating the central noradrenergic system. We draw an analogy between mental disorder and Parkinson's disease, where alterations of the cholinergic system modulate existing parkinsonian symptoms, although they do not in themselves cause the symptoms. The cholinergic system may play a similar modulating role in affective disorders.

In discussing biological theories of schizophrenia, we have formulated a two factor theory of this disorder. We proposed that one feature of this model might involve the balance of dopaminergic and cholinergic functions, rather than dopamine levels alone. Finally, we suggested that the dopaminergic system might play a secondary modulating role in schizophrenia, rather than being its primary cause.

References

Davis, J.M. and Janowsky, D.S.: Amphetamine and methylphenidate psychosis. In Frontiers in Catecholamine Research, ed. by E. Usdin and S. Snyder, pp. 977-987, Pergamon Press, Great Britain, 1973.

El-Yousef, M.K., Janowsky, D.S., Davis, J.M. and Sekerke, H.J.: Reversal of antiparkinsonian drug toxicity by physostigmine: A controlled study. Am. J. Psych. 130: 141-145, 1973.

Janowsky, D.S., El-Yousef, M.K., Davis, J.M. and Sekerke, H.J.: A cholinergic-adrenergic hypothesis of mania and depression. Lancet 2: 632-635, 1972.

Janowsky, D.S., El-Yousef, M.K. and Davis, J.M.: Provocation of schizophrenic symptoms by intravenous administration of methylphenidate. Arch. Gen. Psych. 28: 185-190, 1973a.

Janowsky, D.S., El-Yousef, M.K., Davis, J.M. and Sekerke, H.J.: Antagonistic effects of physostigmine in methylphenidate in man. Am. J. Psych. 130: 12, 1973b.

Janowsky, D.S., El-Yousef, M.K., Davis, J.M. and Sekerke, H.J.: Parasympathetic suppression of manic symptoms by physostigmine. Arch. Gen. Psych. 28: 542-547, 1973c.

Meltzer, H.: Serum creatine phosphokinase and serum aldolase levels in acutely psychotic patients. In Enzymology in the Practice of Laboratory Medicine, ed. by P. Blume and E.F. Freier, pp. 351-379, Academic Press, New York, 1974.

Meltzer, H., Grinspoon, L. and Shader, R.: Serum creatinine kinase activity in acute schizophrenic patients and their relatives. Comp. Psych. 11: 552-558, 1970.

Murphy, D.L. and Wyatt, R.J.: Reduced monoamine oxidase activity in blood platelets from schizophrenic patients. Nature 238: 225-226, 1972.

Robinson, D.S., Davis, J.M., Nies, A., Ravaris, C.L. and Sylvester, D.: Relation of sex and aging to monoamine oxidase activity of human brain, plasma and platelets. Arch. Gen. Psych. 24: 536-539, 1971.

Scheel-Krüger, J.: Comparative studies of various amphetamine analogues demonstrating different interactions with the metabolism of catecholamines in the brain. Eur. J. Pharmacol. 14: 47-49, 1971.

Neurotransmitter Balances Regulating Behavior,
edited and published by E.F. Domino and
J.M. Davis, Ann Arbor, © 1975

REBOUND PHENOMENA IN MANIC PATIENTS FOLLOWING PHYSOSTIGMINE: TOWARDS AN UNDERSTANDING OF THE AMINERGIC MECHANISMS UNDERLYING AFFECTIVE DISORDERS

Baron Shopsin, David Janowsky,
John Davis and Samuel Gershon

Dr. Shopsin and Dr. Gershon are with the Department of Psychiatry, Neuropsychopharmacology Research Unit, New York University School of Medicine, New York, New York.
Dr. Davis is at the Illinois State Psychiatric Institute.
Dr. Janowsky is with the Department of Psychiatry, University of California at San Diego, La Jolla, California.

It has recently been proposed that central cholinergic factors may play a role in the etiology of affective disorders (Janowsky *et al.*, 1972a). Specifically, a balance between central cholinergic and adrenergic neurotransmitter activity in specified brain areas which regulate affect may be involved, with depression being a disease of cholinergic dominance and mania being one of adrenergic dominance. Physostigmine is a reversible cholinesterase inhibitor which increases central acetylcholine levels and thus disturbs central cholinergic-adrenergic balance. This drug has been used to antagonize or neutralize mania as well as euphoric symptoms related to other illnesses, and to cause depression, and has been shown to have effects opposite to those occurring in situations where adrenergic activation occurs (Janowsky *et al.*, 1972a,b, 1973a).

Extending this investigational lead, our departments jointly undertook to explore the effects of physostigmine in severely disturbed manic patients. Two distinct phases of clinical change occurred in all patients during physostigmine administration, as well as a third, post-physostigmine phase, referred to as "rebounding," or compensatory phenomena. This latter phase occurred after the direct effects of this drug had worn off. The present findings of rebounding following physostigmine administration may contribute to our understanding of the aminergic mechanisms underlying the affective illnesses. More than the observed clinical changes occurring during physostigmine administration, the findings may provide an index of the specific adrenergic-dopaminergic-cholinergic imbalance present in a given patient manifesting one of the affective illnesses.

Methods

The subjects included 3 male patients, hospitalized at the Neuropsychopharmacology Research Unit, New York University Medical Center. All 3 patients were in the acute manic phase of cyclic (bipolar) manic-depressive illness. Baseline severity was moderate to severe. Diagnosis and assessment of baseline psychopathology were determined by unanimous decision among 4 psychiatrists.

Each patient was pretreated with methylscopolamine bromide, 1.0 mg, administered i.m. An i.v. infusion of 5% D and W was started 30 min after methylscopolamine administration. Physostigmine or placebo was given piggyback through the D and W tubing, each dose of physostigmine containing either 0.25 mg or 0.50 mg of physostigmine. Physostigmine was given after a varying number of placebo injections and, once started, given at 5 min intervals. The psychiatrists rating the patient were blind as to the time when physostigmine was started. Physicians rated the patients as to affect, mood, and behavior. Clinical notes were taken throughout the experiment. Total dosage of physostigmine differed in all 3 patients, ranging from 3.0 to 6.0 mg total dosage. All patients were given placebo injections following the last active dosage of physostigmine. Pulse and blood pressure were monitored throughout, and the patient was constantly monitored on an EKG. As the study had been designed and consistent with previous experiments by this group, all participants were blind as to injection sequence of active drug substituting for placebo. Although rating scales were used (as has been previously described), clinical notes were taken throughout and the results to be presented in the following section represent information gleaned from both sources.

Results

All 3 patients, irrespective of different overall dosage of physostigmine given, tended to show two rather distinct phases throughout the run itself, as well as a third post-physostigmine stage, to which we shall refer as "rebounding."

In phase 1, all patients experienced, to varying degrees, sedation, drowsiness, a desire but inability to sleep, some dysarthria and mild slurring of speech (2 patients), confusion and difficulty in concentrating. A reduction in spontaneous speech and activity was apparent during this time. Two patients initially described feelings of comfort/relaxation; this subjective comfort dissipated in both cases.

During this phase, it appeared that flight of ideas, rambling, tangentiality, irritability, and cheerfulness were attenuated, with diminished verbal aggressivity and grandiose ideation. Scores for rated molecular items, including talking, grandiosity, flight of ideas, cheerfulness, and activity, accordingly fell. However, speech, like activity, was not spontaneous. The delusional quality of manic psychopathology was not basically altered; prompting or provoking any patient resulted in a reappearance (sometimes full blown) of manic ideation. The severity of manic symptoms reappearing on provocation depended obviously upon the observed degree of anergia. All patients spontaneously stated that they were eventually "talked out" and did not want to be bothered; they all requested to be left alone. This was accompanied by an ill-definable malaise and nausea; vomiting did not occur. Apathy and anergia were apparent but no patient became depressed.

Toward the end of the physostigmine run and always past the 2 mg mark, all patients showed irritability, sweating, and even agitation; this last, *i.e.*, agitation, with marked restlessness, was quite apparent in two patients (phase 2).

The most striking and salient features emerging from this study are the appearance of "rebounding," *i.e.*, clear-cut changes in clinical state taking place 2 hrs after the last physostigmine injection. In two patients, a marked exacerbation or intensification of the manic state was observed; in one of these individuals a psychotomimetic or activating effect occurred in the form of primary process behavior, which was not observed previously to nor since that time in this patient. In a third patient, almost total normalization of mood, affect, ideation, and behavior occurred; normalization was achieved to the extent that all raters judged the patient to be "dischargeable" at that time. These rebounding phenomena were transient in nature, *i.e.*, they all occurred 2 hrs after the last physostigmine injection and lasted for 3 to 4 hrs thereafter, with a return to baseline psychopathology at approximately 6 hrs following the last physostigmine injection.

Discussion

The most striking feature characterizing phase 1 was a reduction in spontaneous speech and activity, apparently secondary to a drug-induced anergic state. Symptoms of drowsiness, confusion, difficulty in concentration, and malaise in our patients suggest some lack of specificity. The marked anxiety, agitation, and severe malaise ensuing in phase 2 would support this assumption. The delusional quality of the manic state was largely unaltered. The exact clinical significance of these changes with regard to the underlying manic state has been questioned (Carroll *et al.*, 1973). Differences in data interpretation exist among our group, and these will be discussed in greater detail elsewhere.

The interpretation of the "rebounding" phenomena and their implication with regard to adrenergic-dopaminergic-cholinergic control mechanisms in affective disorders appear highly relevant with regard to a previous hypothesis (Janowsky *et al.*, 1972a). In the two patients whose mania intensified, a post-physostigmine adrenergic hypersensitivity or cholinergic insensitivity (underactivity), or possibly a combination of both, may be involved. A relative acetylcholine imbalance (reduction) may occur when the physostigmine has been metabolized away about 2 hrs after its administration. Alternatively, the absence of acetylcholine 2 hrs after central flooding with physostigmine may bring about increased adrenergic receptor sensitivity or hyperreactivity to norepinephrine. A compensatory overactivity or increase in activity of the adrenergic system after the disappearance of physostigmine would be consistent with this line of reasoning. In that manic individual whose psychopathology in phase 3 became more activated and who perhaps showed psychotomimetic effects, hypersensitivity or an otherwise relative preponderance of the dopaminergic system may be etiopathogenic. Such a line of reasoning would be consistent with the notion that schizophrenia represents an oversensitivity or abnormal sensitivity of the dopaminergic system, as reported by us and others (Angrist *et al.*, 1973; Janowsky *et al.*, 1973a). With regard to the manic patient who became normalized about 2 hrs following physostigmine infusion and who stayed that way over the next several hours, the following possibilities may be considered.

1. A dose-related phenomenon.
2. A slow egress of physostigmine from brain.
3. A post-physostigmine abnormal sensitivity to acetylcholine.

Consistent with this last would be a post-physostigmine depletion hypersensitivity. Relevant to the dose-related phenomenon is the fact that this patient was given 6 mg of physostigmine, which was more than any of the other patients had received.

Similar rebounding, reflecting endogenous compensatory phenomena, has been documented in animal studies (Janowsky *et al.*, 1973b). Indeed, when physostigmine is administered to rats, one sees, several hours later, an increase in psychomotor activity probably related to an increase in dopaminergic or noradrenergic function (Fibiger et al., 1970, 1971). Ho et al. (1971) have demonstrated a time course-related increase of cholineacetylase activity following intraventricular norepinephrine administration to rats. These rebound compensatory findings can thus be shown on an enzymatic as well as a behavioral level.

The relevant implications of the post-physostigmine rebounding may be that such clinical change can be used as a clinical marker/index of the specific aminergic imbalance characterizing baseline psychopathology in a given patient with mania or depression. Whereas clinical change during physostigmine administration would suggest that an initial adrenergic-cholinergic imbalance exists, the exact nature of this imbalance is not known. It would seem that the specific nature of the balance between adrenergic and cholinergic activity would differ from one individual to another within the same polar phase of an affective disorder. For example, the manic phase of cyclic manic-depressive illness may be due to noradrenergic overactivity or, alternatively, to cholinergic underactivity. In either case, clinical symptoms would reflect noradrenergic dominance. Thus, 2 manic individuals with the same severity of baseline psychopathology may differ with regard to their adrenergic-cholinergic imbalance. The nature of the post-physostigmine rebounding may characterize the specific amine most likely responsible for the presenting abnormal affective state. A patient with only minor elevation of norepinephrine, but with marked acetylcholine depletion may, after a physostigmine run, show a normalization of the manic state as a result of depletion hypersensitivity of cholinergic neurons. Alternatively, a manic patient with similar baseline pathology, but with norepinephrine activity markedly high may, after physostigmine, show an aggravation or intensification of manic symptoms due to even greater adrenergic dominance as a result of rebounding or compensatory phenomena following the fall in acetylcholine.

This apparent endogenous compensatory phenomenon, therefore, occurring after the exogenous administration of a drug may, by the very clinical nature of the rebounding, provide an index of the specific amine responsible for a presenting clinical affective illness.

Our findings of a rebound-activating psychotomimetic effect, along with an intensification of manic hyperactivity, may suggest that dopamine is one of the neurotransmitters involved in clinically characterizing affective illness, and may provide a relevant link in our understanding of that interface between schizo-affective illness, excited type, and the manic phase of manic-depressive disorder. There is an increasing body of evidence linking central dopaminergic hyperactivity with animal stereotypy and some forms of human psychoses. A group of drugs which may be loosely termed as dopamine agonists induce animal stereotypy (Randrup and Munkvad, 1967, 1970; Willner _et al._, 1970) and have been shown to be capable of causing psychotic states in man (Connell, 1958; Rylander, 1969; Spensley and Rockwell, 1972; Strian _et al._, 1972), which bear a close resemblance to some forms of schizophrenia (Connell, 1958; Ellinwood, 1967; Angrist and Gershon, 1970). These "dopaminergic drugs" include apomorphine, levodopa, amphetamine, phenmetrazine, methylphenidate, and cocaine, all of which enhance central dopaminergic activity by different mechanisms (Glowinski _et al._, 1966; Snyder _et al._, 1970; Scheel-Krüger, 1972). Some of these drugs can also intensify or aggravate schizophrenic psychopathology (Angrist _et al._, 1973). A further implication of a relationship between central dopaminergic activity and psychoses is suggested by the fact that neuroleptic drugs which block central dopaminergic receptors (Nyback and Sedvall, 1969; Andén, 1970) also block drug-induced animal stereotypy (Andén, 1970; Ho _et al._, 1971) and have proved efficacious against both naturally-occurring psychotic states and human stimulant psychoses (Angrist and Gershon, 1972).

Extending previous hypotheses, we now propose that an imbalance among adrenergic-dopaminergic-cholinergic central neurotransmitters may be responsible for psychotic symptoms, including mania, depression, and schizo-affective psychoses, as well as other forms of schizophrenia. The relative preponderance of a specific neurotransmitter or, in some instances, 2 neurotransmitters would result in the presenting clinical picture. As reflected in figure 1, depression would result from a preponderance of cholinergic activity, mania in its classic form would be an illness of increased adrenergic tone and schizophrenia would be a disease in which dopaminergic activity (or overactivity) is preponderant. A relative preponderance of both dopamine and norepinephrine activity over cholinergic tone would result in symptoms of both mania and schizophrenia, and the clinical "schizo-affective" picture would be dominanted by symptoms reflecting the relative degree of either dopaminergic or noradrenergic overactivity. Similarly, the depressed phase of schizo-affective illness would reflect both enhanced dopaminergic and cholinergic tone. The diagnostic dilemma in clinically differentiating mania and schizo-affective illness as well as changing clinical pictures in the same individual over time (including drug ingestion), becomes more readily understandable.

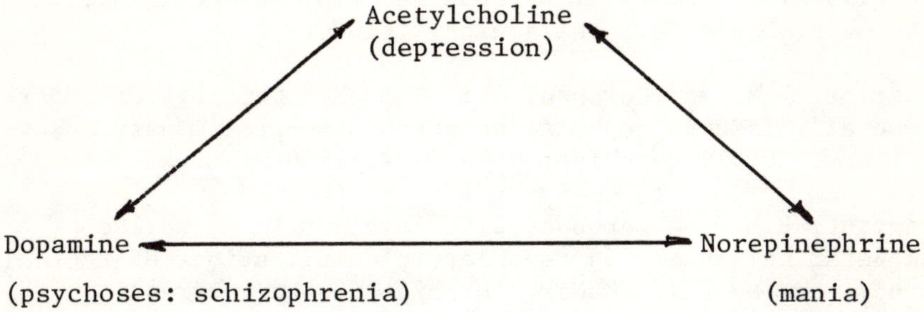

Fig. 1. Model proposing that an imbalance among adrenergic-dopaminergic-cholinergic central neurotransmitters may be responsible for psychotic symptoms, including mania, depression, and schizo-affective psychoses, as well as other forms of schizophrenia. Depression would result from a preponderance of cholinergic activity, mania from a preponderance of adrenergic activity, and schizophrenia from a preponderance of dopaminergic activity. Imbalance of two central neurotransmitters leads to combined symptoms.

Acknowledgements

This work was supported by USPHS Grants MH-17436 and MH-04669.

References

Andén, N.E.: Pharmacological and anatomical implications of induced abnormal movements with L-DOPA. In L-DOPA and Parkinsonism, ed. by A. Barbeau and F.H. McDowell, pp. 132-143, F.A. Davis Co., Philadelphia, 1970.

Angrist, B.M. and Gershon, S.: The phenomenology of experimentally induced amphetamine psychosis--preliminary observations. Biol. Psychiat. 2: 95-107, 1970.

Angrist, B.M. and Gershon, S.: Psychiatric sequellae of amphetamine abuse. In Psychiatric Complications of Medical Drugs, ed. by R.I. Shader, pp. 175-199, Raven Press, New York, 1972.

Angrist, B., Sathananthan, G. and Gershon, S.: Behavioral effects of L-DOPA in schizophrenic patients. Psychopharmacologia 31: 1-12, 1973.

Carroll, B.J., Frazer, A., Schless, A. and Mendels, J.: Cholinergic reversal of manic symptoms. Lancet 1: 427-428, 1973.

Connell, P.H.: Amphetamine Psychosis. Maudsley Monographs No. 5, Oxford University Press, 1958.

Ellinwood, E.H., Jr.: Amphetamine psychosis. I. Description of the individuals and process. J. Nerv. Ment. Dis. 144: 273-283, 1967.

Fibiger, H.C., Lytle, L.D. and Campbell, B.A.: Cholinergic modulation of adrenergic arousal in the developing rat. J. Comp. Physiol. Psychol. 72: 344-349, 1970.

Fibiger, H.C., Lynch, G. and Cooper. H.P.: A biphasic action of central cholinergic stimulation on behavioral arousal in the rat. Psychopharmacologia 20: 366-382, 1971.

Glowinski, J., Axelrod, J. and Iverson, L.L.: Regional studies of catecholamines in rat brain. IV. Effect of drugs on the disposition and metabolism of H^3-norepinephrine and H^3-dopamine. J. Pharmacol. Exp. Ther. 153: 30-41, 1966.

Ho, A.K., Singer, G. and Gershon, S.: Biochemical evidence of adrenergic interaction with cholinergic function in the central nervous system of the rat. I. Effect of norepinephrine. Psychopharmacologia 21: 238-246, 1971.

Janowsky, D.S., El-Yousef, M.K., Davis, J.M. and Sekerke, H.J.: A cholinergic-adrenergic hypothesis of mania and depression. Lancet 2: 632-635, 1972a.

Janowsky, D.S., El-Yousef, M.K., Davis, J.M. and Sekerke, H.J.: Cholinergic antagonism of methylphenidate-induced stereotyped behavior. Psychopharmacologia 27: 295-303, 1972b.

Janowsky, D.S., El-Yousef, M.H., Davis, J.M. and Sekerke, H.J.: Provocation of schizophrenic symptoms by intravenous administration of methylphenidate. Arch. Gen. Psychiat. 28: 185-191, 1973a.

Janowsky, D.S., El-Yousef, M.K., Davis, J.M. and Sekerke, H.J.: Parasympathetic suppression of manic symptoms by physostigmine. Arch. Gen. Psychiat. 28: 542-547, 1973b.

Nyback, H. and Sedvall, G.: Regional accumulation of catecholamines formed from tyrosine-^{14}C in rat brain: Effect of chlorpromazine. Europ. J. Pharmacol. 4: 245-252, 1969.

Randrup, A. and Munkvad, I.: Stereotyped activities produced by amphetamine in several animal species and man. Psychopharmacologia 11: 300-310, 1967.

Randrup, A. and Munkvad, I.: Biochemical, anatomical and psychological investigation of stereotyped behavior induced by amphetamines. In Amphetamines and Related Compounds, ed. by E. Costa and S. Garattini, pp. 695-713, Raven Press, New York, 1970.

Rylander, G.: Clinical and medico-criminological aspects of addiction to central stimulating drug. In Abuse of Central Stimulants, ed. by F. Sjoqvist and M. Tattie, pp. 251-273, Raven Press, New York, 1969.

Scheel-Krüger, J.: Behavioral and biochemical comparison of amphetamine derivatives, cocaine, benztropine and tricyclic anti-depressant drugs. Europ. J. Pharmacol. 18: 63-73, 1972.

Snyder, S.H., Taylor, K.M., Coyle, J.T. and Meyerkoff, J.L.: The role of brain dopamine in behavioral regulation and the actions of psychotropic drugs. Amer. J. Psychiat. 127: 199-207, 1970.

Spensley, J. and Rockwell, D.A.: Psychosis during methylphenidate abuse. New Eng. J. Med. 286: 880-881, 1972.

Strian, F., Micheler, E. and Benkert, O.: Tremor inhibition in Parkinson syndrome after apomorphine administration under L-DOPA and decarboxylase inhibition basic therapy. Pharmakopsychiat. 5: 198-205, 1972.

Willner, J.H., Samach, M., Angrist, B.M., Wallach, M.B. and Gershon, S.: Drug-induced stereotyped behavior and its antagonism in dogs. Comm. Behav. Biol. 5: 135-149, 1970.

Neurotransmitter Balances Regulating Behavior,
edited and published by E.F. Domino and
J.M. Davis, Ann Arbor, © 1975

ADRENERGIC AND CHOLINERGIC FACTORS IN EXTRAPYRAMIDAL DISORDERS

William E. Fann
Baylor College of Medicine
Houston, Texas

C. Raymond Lake
Duke University Medical Center
Durham, North Carolina

Gerald M. McKenzie
Burroughs Wellcome Laboratories
Research Triangle, North Carolina

Current theories of drug-induced dyskinesias posit a putative imbalance between CNS acetylcholine (ACh) and dopamine (DA) neuronal mechanisms, with a consequent dominance of dopamine activity (Fann et al., 1974). It is thought that chronic administration of neuroleptics blocks postsynaptic DA receptor sites and causes either a "functional" denervation-type hypersensitivity of these neurons or, through an undefined feedback mechanism, stimulates excessive synthesis and release of DA by the presynaptic neuron. In this manner, a hyperdopaminergic state is developed which results in manifestations of tardive dyskinesia. Such a state would be similar to the postulated mechanism in the heredodegenerative disease, Huntington's Chorea (HC). In HC there is a diminution of striatal dopaminergic neurons with a normal amount of total DA, suggesting a hyperdopaminergic condition appearing clinically as hyperkinesis (Klawans and Rubovitz, 1972).

We have conducted a series of studies testing the clinical efficacy of adrenergic and cholinergic compounds on meliorating symptoms of various movement disorders. This is a report of some of these investigations.

Methods

Groups of subjects manifesting various extrapyramidal disorders were administered the cholinergic substances physostigmine and deanol (2-methylaminoethanol) and the adrenergic dopaminergic substances methylphenidate and amantadine.

Rigid Huntington's Disease. Three sisters, ages 24, 28

and 32 years, all chronically hospitalized in a state mental institution with varying degrees of advanced mental and physical deterioration secondary to a chronic degenerative nervous system disease, were transferred to the Duke University Hospital Clinical Research Unit. These patients all showed early in the course of their condition varying degrees of hyperkinesis, considered typical of Huntington's Disease. The onset of rigidity came gradually and proceeded at varying rates. Over a period of 18 months, during which time they were followed by a faculty neurologist, the youngest developed the greatest degree of rigidity. On the basis of this evidence, the patients' inability to perform saccadic eye movements or respond to caloric vestibular tests, pervasive plastic rigidity, declining or absent hyperkinesis and mental deterioration, the neurologist made the diagnosis of rigid Huntington's disease. All three patients were receiving anticonvulsant medication as a result of seizure histories. The youngest demonstrated the most pronounced rigidity and mental and physical deterioration, while the oldest was the most intact. The elder, though showing generalized plastic rigidity, evinced moderate to mild hyperkinesia of the face, diaphragm, arms, and neck. This constituted a diminution of the degree noted on the initial examination 18 months previous.

After careful physical examination and laboratory results revealed no contraindication for physostigmine treatment, each patient was premedicated with the quaternary anticholinergic, methylscopolamine, 0.25 mg s.c., a compound previously used in similar trials (Duvoisin, 1967; Klawans and Rubovitz, 1972). This was followed by physostigmine, 30 μg/kg i.m. Neurological examinations were performed by two raters one day before and immediately before physostigmine injection, 30 and 90 min, and one day after injection, using Crane's neurological rating scale.

Hyperkinetic Huntington's Disease. Three subjects, two male and one female, ages 43, 52 and 50, all chronically hospitalized in a state mental hospital with established diagnoses of Huntington's disease were given physical examinations and laboratory screen including EKG and found to have no contraindications to physostigmine. Each was administered physostigmine, 40 μg/kg i.v. in amount and method previously demonstrated to provoke changes in the involuntary movements of Huntington's disease (Aquilonius and Sjöstrom, 1971; Klawans and Rubovitz, 1972) and Parkinsonism (Duvoisin, 1967). The injections were given slowly over a period of 3 to 5 min per individual. Peripheral cholinergic action was blocked by concomitant administration of methylscopolamine, a quaternary anticholinergic salt which does not cross the blood-brain barrier, mixed in the syringe with the physostigmine. The dose of this agent ranged from .25-.5 mg, according to the dose of physostigmine. In this manner, the peripheral effects of physostigmine were reduced without interfering with its enhancement of central acetylcholine activity. All three subjects were maintained on their phenothiazine medication.

Each subject was videotaped immediately before being given the physostigmine, 45 min and 24 hr after injection. The videotaping procedures for all subjects were uniform in all respects. Each subject was allowed an adjustment period of approximately 10 min in the room and was then directed through a standard examination routine previously described (Fann *et al*., 1972). The taped sequences, 10 min per subject, were re-run randomly and rated on a blind basis by two faculty neurologists, who assessed symptoms on a global estimation of severity on the following five parameters: hand-fingers, feet, head, mouth-lip, tongue. The tapes were played again for recheck at the request of the raters during their individual sessions. The estimation of severity of the body part dyskinesia was made on a 100 point scale, with 0 reflecting absence of movement and 100 the most severe the neurologist had ever seen.

Tardive Dyskinesia. In a trial of methylphenidate a group of 30 hospitalized patients, diagnosed independently by other clinicans as having tardive dyskinesia, were taken into the study. EKG, physical examination, blood studies, and urinalysis were performed before and after the treatment. Blood pressure and pulse readings were recorded. Patients were housed on their regular treatment wards and were escorted once a week to the office of the rater, where they were examined 10 min each and rated on Crane's neurological scale. This method has proven highly reliable in our laboratory. Nurses' Observation Scale for In-patient Evaluation (Nosie-30) forms were completed weekly by the ward staff. Global ratings were made from global reports systematically collected from members of the ward staff and other observers (e.g., vocational rehabilitation counselors occupational therapists) of the patients' overall functioning and ability to carry out activities of daily living. Videotapes were made of each subject before, during, and after treatment, re-run in random sequence, and rated blind. Half the subjects were randomly placed in the placebo group and half received the active drug. All subjects began by receiving 20 mg of methylphenidate per day (or its placebo equivalent) and the dosage increased for each patient by equal weekly increments to a maximum of 80 mg/day. At the end of six weeks the two groups were crossed over. All subjects continued to receive the prescribed neuroleptics, 200-800 mg of chlorpromazine a day or its equivalent. Phenothiazines were the only neuroleptics used.

In the physostigmine trial, seven chronic state mental hospital patients, six female and one male, all diagnosed by two raters as having tardive dyskinesia, were accepted for study after providing informed consent and after physical examination, clinical history and laboratory screen, including EKG, revealed no contraindication to the medication. All carried a diagnosis of schizophrenia, though organic brain disease could not be ruled out in three. The patients ranged in age from 55 to 70 years. In the past each had been treated at various times with several phenothiazines, haloperidol, and antiparkinson agents, but none was receiving medication other than phenothiazines at the time of the study. Because several subjects had multiple past hospital admissions, including two at hospitals from which complete records were not available, the total hospitalization time could not be accurately tabulated. Nevertheless, all of the subjects had been hospitalized for a total of at least three years and had been on long-term neuroleptic therapy. Each was administered physostigmine in the amount and by the method described above and rated in the same manner as the Huntington's Disease patients.

In a trial of deanol, six subjects diagnosed independently by other clinicians as having tardive dyskinesia were given deanol in an open study, 500 mg/day in divided doses orally. All subjects were screened for history of sensitivity to stimulant compounds and blood pressure determinations, standing and supine, were elicited four times daily. Each was rated immediately before, 24 hr and three days after starting the deanol on a global estimation of diminishing symptomatology.

<u>Drug-induced Parkinsonism</u>. Forty-one hospitalized subjects, 21 males and 20 females, diagnosed by two clinicians as having drug-induced parkinsonism, were taken into the study after physical examination, clinical history and laboratory screens, including EKG, revealed no contraindication to a stimulant-type antiparkinson agent. The ages ranged from 17 to 72 years, with an average of 43 years. All developed drug-induced extrapyramidal symptoms while being treated with anti-psychotic medication for illnesses diagnosed as follows: schizophrenia (N=36), senile psychosis (N=2), manic-depressive psychosis (N=1), postpartum psychosis (N=1), chronic brain syndrome associated with syphilis (N-1). Pregnant females and patients with Parkinson's disease were excluded from the study. The patients were allocated at random to two groups (a→s) and (s→a). Group (a→s)

received trihexiphenidyl as coded medication for two weeks; Group (s→a) received amantadine as coded medication for two weeks. Severity of parkinsonism and side effects were measured at baseline (just before coded medication) and at examinations scheduled for the first, third, seventh, tenth and fourteenth day of medication. After 14 days, placebo was substituted for coded medication. Those patients in whom significant parkinsonism occurred on placebo were given the alternate to the first coded medication for a second two week period, during which they were scheduled for examination as before. Both periods of coded medication were double blind. The placebo period was single blind.

Practical exigencies precluded strict adherence to the planned examination schedule. Examinations following within the day of the specified time were accepted in lieu of missing examinations. Some examinations were missed, but sufficient data were obtained for a meaningful analysis. The severity of parkinsonism was rated on the Simpson-Angus rating scale of each examination. The following signs were rated, 0-4, in increasing order of severity:

Gait
Arm-dropping
Shoulder shaking
Elbow rigidity
Waist rigidity
Leg pendulousness
Glabella tap
Tremor
Salivation

Eight treatment-emergent parameters were scored 0-3, in increasing order of severity at each examination:

Dry mouth
Visual disturbance
Urinary hesitancy
Hearing disturbance
Restlessness
Confusion
Agitation
Tardive Dyskinesia

Acute Drug-induced Dyskinesia and Dystonia. Ten subjects with acute drug-induced dystonia, all hospitalized for varying diagnoses of psychosis were accepted for the study. All had been treated acutely with large doses of neuroleptics and variously manifested occulogyric crises, torticollis, trunkal torsion, and protrusion of the tongue; a dyskinetic patient showed clenching of the jaw, shifting of the body weight from one foot to the other, and aimless movement of the hands within several days of starting neuroleptic treatment. Each patient was given methylphenidate, 25-50 mg in a slow i.v. injection. Each was administered at least 25 mg, but not all subjects required 50 mg for relief of symptoms. Another group of 10 subjects showing the same symptoms was given diphenhydramine, 10-50 mg i.m. Another five subjects with movements more characteristic of akathisia than dyskinesia were given methylphenidate, 25-50 mg i.v. and then started on trihexyphenidyl, 8 mg/day.

Animal Study. To test the development of tolerance to the chlorpromazine-induced increase in dopamine turnover, adult male Sprague-Dawley rats were given chlorpromazine daily. Various groups were sacrificed after one day, four days, and 10 days. Each was given H^3-tyrosine, 500 μc/kg (specific activity - 30-50 c/mmol), i.p. The animal was sacrificed one hr later, using fluothane. The brain material was assayed for tritiated dopamine, tritiated acidic catechols, and total tritium. Statistical significance was calculated using Student's t test.

Results

Rigid Huntington's Disease. In none of the three propositi were any significant changes found in either the general neurological status or in the rigidity and involuntary movement of arms, legs, neck, or trunk of the patient. There was nearly complete inter-rater agreement on all measurements. There were some side effects including vomiting, diarrhea, increased bowel activity, and measured salivation.

Hyperkinetic Huntington's Disease. All three subjects showed some alterations in all of the parameters at 45 min and at 24 hr. These findings were inconsistent, however, and no definite pattern of response could be discerned from these data. The patients did not subjectively change (i.e., they reported no mood alterations from their pre-drug condition) at any time following the physostigmine. The objective ratings from the videotapes were corroborated by the global impressions from the staff. Side effects included some nausea, abdominal cramping, and tension.

Tardive Dyskinesia. In the methylphenidate trials, 17 of the 30 subjects completed the 12 weeks of the study. Of the remaining 13 patients, five displayed an increase in psychiatric symptoms, becoming unruly or hyperactive. These five were removed from the methylphenidate treatment. Eight others were removed for administrative reasons (e.g., discharged at family requests or transferred to other units). Seventeen who completed the study were compared on several ratings between methylphenidate and placebo.

The Nosie scales for those patients remaining on the study showed no significant changes. No differences were found from serial assessment of the videotape. The weekly blind ratings showed no definite or consistent changes in the neurological symptomatology for either group at any time. On the global weekly neurological ratings by the nurse and ward staff, six patients showed some increase in hyperkinesia, eight showed no change, and three were judged to have improved while taking methylphenidate. These three became able to feed themselves, tie their shoe strings, carry cafeteria trays, and dress themselves. This improvement was lost when methylphenidate was withdrawn.

Side effects included a transient (five day) rise of 20 mm Hg in the systolic blood pressure of one patient, transient moderate (trace-2+) protein urea in five women patients, and EKG changes that had no corresponding clinical symptoms in three.

In the physostigmine study (tables 1, 2, 3) some decrease in the severity of the movements could be detected after 45 min. In the five of seven subjects who showed abnormal tongue movements, all five were judged by at least one rater to have improved; in three there was complete inter-rater agreement. This decrease in comparison to control was significant by t test ($P < 0.025$). Six of seven subjects showed abnormal mouth-lip movements. Three of the six were rated as improved. All seven of the subjects showed involuntary hand-finger movements. Only two of these were rated as displaying less hand-finger movement after 45 min lapse time. The changes were non-significant for the group (t test). At 24 hr, tongue movement was decreased in five subjects with highly significant ($P < 0.0005$) inter-rater agreement in all. Mouth-lip motion was decreased in five of the six ($P < 0.0005$). Six of the seven showing abnormal hand-finger motion were given lower values after 24 hr ($P < 0.01$). In the head and feet parameters, abnormal movements were not present in enough of the subjects and, where present, were of insignificant magnitude to make a statistical comparison.

Side effects of the physostigmine included mild abdominal cramps in three subjects, acute moderate diarrhea in two, and nausea in two, all of which abated within two hr after the injection. No changes in alertness or psychopathology were noted in any of the subjects. A several week follow-up of each subject revealed no side effects or sequelae related to the physostigmine.

Table 1

Effect of physostigmine on tongue movements in tardive dyskinesia

Patient	45 min	24 hr
1	0.4	0.4
	0.5	0.3
3	0.7	0.7
	1.3	0.3
4	0.2	0.4
	0.5	0.5
5	1.0	0.9
	0.9	0.4
6	0.8	0.7
	0.8	0.4
	P <0.025	P <0.005

Values given by two raters are expressed as ratio of drug/control values at 45 min and 24 hr after i.v. physostigmine. P is in comparison to control (t test).

Table 2

Effect of physostigmine on mouth-lip movements in tardive dyskinesia

Patient	45 min	24 hr
1	0.7	0.7
	1.0	1.0
3	1.0	0.9
	1.7	0.3
4	0.3	0.5
	0.1	0.4
5	1.0	0.8
	1.2	0.2
6	0.8	0.5
	0.5	0.2
9	0.8	0.5
	0.8	0.5
	N.S.	P <0.001

Values given by two raters are expressed as ratio of drug/control values at 45 min and 24 hr after i.v. physostigmine. P in comparison to control (t test). N.S. = nonsignificant (t test).

Table 3

Effects of physostigmine on hand-finger movements in tardive dyskinesia

Patient	45 min	24 hr
1	1.0	1.0
	1.3	0.8
2	1.0	0.1
	1.3	0.3
3	0.2	0.2
	1.0	1.0
4	1.0	1.0
	0.5	1.0
5	0.8	0.4
	1.0	0.5
6	0.3	0.1
	0.3	0.1
9	0.7	0.1
	0.5	0.4
	N.S.	P <0.01

Values given by two raters are expressed as ratio of drug/control values at 45 min and 24 hr after i.v. physostigmine. P in comparison to control (t test). N.S. = non-significant (t test).

Drug-induced Parkinsonism. Both the trihexyphenidyl and amantadine were effective treatments for drug-induced parkinsonism. Their efficacies according to our preliminary data were equivalent.

Of patients who completed the second period of coded medication, 20 experienced recurrence of significant parkinsonism on placebo. Of this group, which included 9 of the 20 in the (a→s) group and 11 of the 22 in the (s→a) group, the data elicited by baseline placebo and 14 day examinations on both coded medications were evaluated. Again, in this group the data are consistent, with trihexyphenidyl and amantadine being of equivalent efficacy in treatment of drug-induced parkinsonism.

Side effect incidence was approximately the same for both compounds. Slightly more anticholinergic activity (*i.e.*, dry mouth) was attributable to the trihexyphenidyl than to amantadine. Tardive dyskinesia, seen in three of the subjects who also experienced drug-induced parkinsonism (*i.e.*, cogwheel rigidity), was mildly aggravated by both compounds.

Acute drug-induced dystonia and dyskinesia. The subjects with acute drug-induced dystonia responded equally well to trihexyphenidyl or other atropine-like antiparkinson agents or to methylphenidate. The drug-induced dyskinesia responded inconsistently to either compound. Some of the subjects improved with the trihexyphenidyl and others did not.

Animal Study. In this pilot study, the possibility of the development of tolerance to the chlorpromazine-induced increase in dopamine turnover in rat striatum is suggested (table 4). After one day of chlorpromazine, there was a highly significant increase in tritiated dopamine and tritiated acidic catechols. The values after four and ten days were not significantly elevated over control values, however. After 20 mg of chlorpromazine per kg twice daily for 10 days, the tritiated dopamine values had dropped below normal to a significant degree. The tritiated acetic metabolites were not significantly altered as compared to control.

Discussion

Most treatment of drug-induced extrapyramidal disorders has in some way involved adjustment of CNS dopamine and acetylcholine (Fann *et al.*, 1973). Prange and his coworkers (1973) have shown that compounds which alter CNS serotonin levels also affect some movement disorders. Therapy for drug-induced parkinsonism, a condition supposedly brought about through antagonism of striatal dopaminergic

Table 4

Pilot Study:
Development of tolerance to the chlorpromazine induced increase in dopamine turnover in the rat striatum

Treatment	N	H^3-DA	P	H^3-AC[+]	P	H^3-T	P
Control	13	48,310 ± 1377	-	5914 ± 698	-	363,443 ± 11,913	-
CPZ-20	4	78,597 ± 8420	<0.001	23,475 ± 1832	<0.001	382,339 ± 16,195	N.S.
*CPZ-20-b.i.d.- 4 days	4	60,673 ± 6423	N.S.	16,229 ± 1910	<0.001	383,231 ± 38,550	N.S.
*CPZ-10-b.i.d.- 10 days	3	56,115 ± 7957	N.S.	13,968 ± 2240	<0.01	299,015 ± 18,944	<0.02
*CPZ-20-b.i.d.- 10 days	3	38,595 ± 401	<0.01	7,677 ± 518	N.S.	311,355 ± 16,183	<0.05
*Saline-b.i.d.- 10 days	3	69,513 ± 11,673	N.S.	25,083 ± 4090	0.001	302,129 ± 21,641	<0.05

*Plus CPZ 20 mg/kg
P values using "t" test.
t = Acidic Catechols

systems by the neuroleptics, usually involves administration of an atropine-like agent which lowers striatal acetylcholine activity (Duvoisin, 1967). In normal motor function, a condition of a balance exists between the activity of the dopaminergic and acetylcholine-dependent systems. Drugs which effectively raise the activity of catecholamines will also alleviate parkinsonism, acting putatively by raising the level of dopaminergic activity rather than suppressing acetylcholine. Stimulant compounds, such as amphetamine and methylphenidate, may aggravate the psychiatric symptoms for which the subject is being treated with neuroleptics, and are seldom recommended for long-term therapy. For this reason, agents which suppress acetylcholine are considered the drugs of choice and are most widely used clinically. Our data on the response of tardive dyskinesia to cholinergic agents called the practice into question, however. The possibility that a cholinergic deficit exists in tardive dyskinesia suggests that long-term suppression of acetylcholine-dependent mechanisms may contribute to this condition (Fann et al., 1974). If this is true, then a compound which elevates striatal dopamine levels would be preferable to one which suppresses the acetylcholine system in order to restore balance with the antagonized dopamine systems. This is apparently the mechanism of action of the antiparkinson compound amantadine (Heikkila et al., 1972; Heimans et al., 1972; Herblin, 1972). Though some question remains as to its mechanism of action in man, it is putatively a dopaminergic agent. It would, therefore, restore dopamine mechanisms to activity rather than suppress the relatively healthy acetylcholine-dependent mechanism to reverse the drug-induced parkinsonism.

The finding that methylphenidate increased the symptoms of tardive dyskinesia is consistent with current theories of this condition (Klawans, 1973). TD, according to some theories, is a result of excessive dopamine activity in the striatum. Thus, the neuroleptics block postsynaptic dopamine receptor sites, stimulating an increase in turnover and a subsequent increase in dopamine synthesis, with a possible accompanying functional hypersensitivity of the postsynaptic neuronal receptor site through chronic blocking of the receptor site. Either or both of these conditions (i.e. an excess amount of the transmitter agent or an excessively sensitive receptor site) would result in the postulated hyperdopaminergic state. Our data, however, suggest that a malfunction of acetylcholine-dependent systems may obtain in tardive dyskinesia. Subjects given physostigmine, which acts approximately 2 hrs in man, showed a greater suppression of movement after 24 hrs than at 45 min, a finding which suggests that the systems are not only suppressed but that they may be "revitalized" to function normally for at least a short time.

Our finding that a putative oral cholinergic agent, deanol, also suppresses the movement of tardive dyskinesia would tend to corroborate this theory and suggest that our approach to the treatment of tardive dyskinesia, through enhancement of striatal acetylcholine, is correct. This also makes good clinical sense, compared to the suggestions that tardive dyskinesia be treated through increasing the dose of the offending neuroleptic (Singer, 1971; Peters et al., 1972; Kazamatsuri et al., 1973). The neuroleptics, by blocking the dopamine receptor sites, will decrease the dopamine effect and thereby suppress tardive dyskinesia. Since these compounds are implicated in the genesis of tardive dyskinesia, however, we would clearly be risking more damage to the insulted neuronal systems rather than relieving the syndrome (Uhrbrand and Faurbye, 1960).

The reversal of acute neuroleptic-induced dystonic conditions and parkinsonism by anticholinergics, amantadine and methylphenidate, suggest that reduced dopamine activity is present in these disorders. These findings are, of course, consistent with current theories of the condition. The fact that acute dyskinesia and akathisia have responded inconsistently to methylphenidate, and may be aggravated by anticholinergic activities, suggests that not all of these conditions are due simply to reduction in dopamine activity, but are due to alterations of acetylcholine as well. Our data on deanol, which acts putatively by increasing synthesis of acetylcholine, infer that this agent may be effective in the treatment of those extrapyramidal disorders related to hypofunction of acetylcholine dependent systems.

The data suggest that both acetylcholine- and dopamine-dependent systems are involved in some extrapyramidal nervous system disorders and give implications for clinical application of these findings.

The data from one pilot study in animals does not, of course, allow firm conclusions to be drawn, though the data on dopamine turnover in animal striatum following chronic chlorpromazine administration suggest that tolerance to chlorpromazine-induced turnover of dopamine does develop. This at least calls into question the hyperdopaminergic theories of tardive dyskinesia and supports our hypothesis that a hypocholinergic defect exists in this condition. We recognize, of course, that further studies are necessary and are proceeding accordingly in our own laboratori

Acknowledgments

The authors are grateful to Bruce Richman and Connie Ramey for technical assistance in the conduct of this work.

References

Aquilonius, J.M. and Sjöstrom, R.: Cholinergic and dopaminergic mechanisms in Huntington's Chorea. Life Sci. 10: 405-414, 1971.

Duvoisin, R.C.: Cholinergic-anticholinergic antagonism in parkinsonism. Arch. Neurol. 17: 124-136, 1967.

Fann, W.E., Davis, J.M. and Janowsky, D.S.: Tardive dyskinesia: Findings in two mental hospital populations. Dis. Nerv. Sys. 33: 182-186, 1972.

Fann, W.E., Davis, J.M. and Wilson, I.C.: Methylphenidate in tardive dyskinesia. Am. J. Psychiat. 130: 922-924, 1973.

Fann, W.E., Lake, C.R., Gerber, C.J. and McKenzie, G.M.: Cholinergic suppression of tardive dyskinesia. Psychopharmacologia 37: 101-107, 1974.

Heikkila, R.E. and Cohen, G.: Evaluation of amantadine as a releasing agent or uptake blocker for H^3-dopamine in rat brain slices. Eur. J. Pharmacol. 20: 156-160, 1972.

Heimans, R.L., Rand, M.J. and Fennessy, M.R.: Effects of amantadine on uptake and release of dopamine by a particulate fraction of rat basal ganglia. J. Pharm. Pharmacol. 24: 875-879, 1972.

Herblin, W.F.: Amantadine and catecholamine uptake. Biochem. Pharmacol. 21: 1993-1995, 1972.

Kazamatsuri, H., Chien, C. and Cole, J.L.: Long-term treatment of tardive dyskinesia with haloperidol and tetrabenazine. Am. J. Psychiat. 130: 479-483, 1973.

Klawans, H.L., Jr. and Rubovitz, R.: Central cholinergic-anticholinergic antagonism in Huntington's Chorea. Neurol. 22: 107-116, 1972.

Klawans, H.L., Jr.: The pharmacology of tardive dyskinesia. Am. J. Psychiat. 130: 82-86, 1973.

Peters, H.A., Daley, R.F. and Sato, S.: Reserpine for tardive dyskinesia. New Engl. J. Med. 286: 106, 1972.

Prange, A.J., Jr., Wilson, I.C., Morris, C.E. and Hall, C.D.: Preliminary experience with tryptophan and lithium in treatment of tardive dyskinesia. Psychopharmacol. Bull. 9: 36-37, 1973.

Singer, K.: Thiopropazate HCl in persistent dyskinesia. Brit. Med. J. 4: 22-25, 1971.

Uhrbrand, L. and Faurbye, A.: Reversible and irreversible dyskinesia after treatment with perphenazine, chlorpromazine, reserpine, and electroconvulsive therapy. Psychopharmacologia 1: 408-418, 1960.

Neurotransmitter Balances Regulating Behavior,
edited and published by E.F. Domino and
J.M. Davis, Ann Arbor, © 1975

DIMETHYLTRYPTAMINE: ITS BIOSYNTHESIS AND POSSIBLE ROLE IN MENTAL DISEASE

Lewis R. Mandel
Department of Biochemistry
Merck Institute for Therapeutic Research
Rahway, New Jersey

The N,N-dimethylindoleamines are hallucinogenic agents. One member of this family of compounds, N,N-dimethyltryptamine (DMT), is a potent psychotogen in man (Szara, 1967; Shulgin, 1970). DMT is a known human hallucinogen for which there is also a biosynthetic mechanism (Axelrod, 1961), and thus it has been the subject of extensive study, with particular emphasis on its possible relationship to schizophrenia. Several groups have reported that DMT is present in elevated levels in blood and urine of some schizophrenic patients (Greenberg, 1973; Narasimhachari et al., 1971a,b; Rosengarten et al., 1970). The DMT precursor, tryptamine, is present in human brain (Saavedra and Axelrod, 1972), elevated urinary tryptamine is found in some schizophrenics (Himwich, 1971) and monoamine oxidase, the principal enzyme for tryptamine degradation, is reduced in the platelets of some patients (Murphy and Wyatt, 1972; Wyatt et al., 1973b). Administration of the amino acid precursors of DMT, methionine and tryptophane, has been found to exacerbate symptomotology in schizophrenic patients under certain circumstances (Kety, 1967). Failure of DMT to produce tolerance and other evidence, even less direct but consistent with DMT being the schizophrenic hallucinogen, have also been outlined previously (Wyatt et al., 1974).

Axelrod (1961) reported on the occurrence of a nonspecific N-methyltransferase which catalyzes the transfer of the methyl group from S-adenosylmethionine (SAM) to the amino group of a variety of indoles and other amines. This enzyme, capable of forming DMT, was found to be present in high content in rabbit lung and has since been reported to occur in smaller amounts in several tissues from laboratory animals and man (Morgan and Mandell, 1969; Heller, 1971; Mandell and Morgan, 1971; Mandel et al., 1972; Narasimhachari et al., 1972; Saavedra and Axelrod, 1972; Thithapandha, 1972; Saavedra et al., 1973; Wyatt et al., 1973c).

In our initial studies, the enzyme (indoleamine-N-methyltransferase) was purified 50-fold from rabbit lung by ammonium sulfate fractionation, chromatography on Sephadex G-150, then DEAE-sephadex A-50 (Mandel et al., 1971). The partially purified enzyme was free of imidazole- and phenethanolamine-N-methyl transferase activities. While it has been reported that serotonin was the best substrate for the enzyme (Axelrod, 1961), N-methyltryptamine (NMT) was found to exhibit an apparent substrate inhibition when present at relatively high concentrations in the _in vitro_ assay and had the lowest Km (5 x 10^{-5}M) among several indoleamines tested.

A number of other tissues were examined for their content of the DMT-forming enzyme using NMT and SAM (methyl ^{14}C) as co-substrates. Enzyme activity, based upon thin layer chromatographic identification of ^{14}C labeled DMT, was found in dialyzed 78,000 x g supernatants of homogenates from rabbit liver and brain, rat liver, and human liver and lung. Only traces of activity (less than 50 cpm in DMT from 500,000 cpm SAM) were found when enzyme preparations from rat, chick or human brain were assayed, in contrast to findings from other laboratories (Mandell and Morgan, 1969; Saavedra _et al._, 1973). In view of the recent reports involving 5-methyl-^{14}C-tetrahydrofolic acid (MTHF) as an alternate methyl donor (Banarjee and Snyder, 1973; Hsu and Mandell, 1973), ^{14}C-MTHF was substituted for SAM in the _in vitro_ assay. No evidence for DMT formation was found using enzyme preparations from brain, heart, lung or liver from the chick, rat, rabbit or man. MTHF did react with NMT to form a radioactive compound recently identified as 2,3,4,9-tetrahydro-2-methyl 1H-pyrido[3,4b] indole (Mandel _et al._, 1974). Our results demonstrate that MTHF cannot substitute for SAM in the biosynthesis of DMT.

The relatively high activity of the enzyme in human lung made it attractive for more detailed studies (Mandel _et al._, 1972). The enzyme is associated with an inhibitor which is removed by dialysis and centrifugation of the tissue extracts. By minor modification of the methods used to assay the rabbit lung enzyme, activity has been found in 13 of 23 human lung post-mortem specimens. No relationship between the occurrence of enzyme activity and the case histories has been noted. The enzyme was purified 25-fold and the ammonium sulfate fractionation and molecular sieve chromatographic properties found to be similar to those of the rabbit enzyme. NMT was found to be the substrate with the lowest Km (2.8 x 10^{-4}M), and products of the methyltransferase, bufotenin, and DMT were inhibitory. DMT was identified as the _in vitro_ reaction product by thin layer chromatography, reverse isotope dilution assay and combined gas-liquid chromatography-mass spectrometry (Walker _et al._, 1972).

To demonstrate the biosynthesis of DMT _in vivo_, rabbits and rats were pre-treated with the monoamine oxidase inhibitor, pheniprazine, and ^{14}C-NMT (25-35 μc; 0.6 mg/kg administered i.v. (Ahn et al., 1973). Five to forty-five minutes later the animals were decapitated and tissues frozen at -196°. ^{14}C-DMT was extracted and quantified by thin layer radiographic or reverse isotope dilution assay. In the rabbit, ^{14}C-DMT was present in highest amounts in lung, decreasing from 10,000 cpm/gm 5 minutes after administration of precursor NMT to below 900 cpm/gm at 45 minutes. This is in accord with the high content of the DMT forming enzyme in rabbit lung. The maximum DMT content in kidney was 3000 cpm/gm; no DMT was found in blood, spleen, liver or brain. When the ^{14}C-NMT was administered intracisternally, trace amounts of ^{14}C-DMT were found in rabbit brain (100-300 cpm/gm). There was no evidence for conversion of ^{14}C-NMT to ^{14}C-DMT in rat lung, liver, kidney, blood or brain.

Preliminary experiments studying the fate of exogenous DMT were carried out in rabbits. ^{14}C labeled DMT (25 μc; 1 mg/kg) was administered i.v. to pheniprazine pretreated animals and 15 or 60 minutes later they were sacrificed. The percent radioactivity as DMT and its major metabolite was determined in various tissues. At the one hour time point less than 25% of the radioactivity remained as DMT in blood, lung, liver and kidney, whereas nearly half the radioactivity in brain was DMT. The radioactive DMT was equally distributed in the hippocampus, median raphé bundle, and cerebellum with frontal lobe. Trace amounts (0.2-1%) of the demethylated compounds, tryptamine and NTM, were found in all tissues. ^{14}C-labeled indoleacetic acid was identified as the major polar metabolite accounting for up to 23% of the radioactivity in the blood. The bulk (30-96%) of the radioactivity appeared in the non-solvent extractable fraction, possibly as indole conjugates. A rapid rate of metabolism of DMT was also observed when mice were given 15 mg/kg DMT i.p. Ten minutes after injection, 2.7-4.6 μg DMT per gm tissue was recovered from liver, lung and brain, but none was recovered 30-240 minutes after injection. Cohen and Vogel (1972) reported a similar pattern of results in rats.

DMT has been reported (Narasimhachari et al., 1971a,b to be present in blood and urine of schizophrenic patients but not normal controls; a rough correlation between the intensity of the symptoms of the disease and urinary DMT levels has been implied. An association of DMT with schizophrenia has also been reported by Rosengarten and co-workers (1970), and Greenberg (1973). Others (Franzen and Gross, 1965; Gross and Franzen, 1965) found that DMT was not unique to schizophrenics. Our experience has indicated that some of the methodology used to analyze DMT in body fluids lacks the appropriate sensitivity and specificity. One of the techniques employed to characterize DMT in the _in vitro_ enzyme studies was combined gas chromatography-mass spectrometry (Walker _et al_., 1972). By modifying this methodology, an isotope dilution assay for DMT in blood, urine and spinal fluid was developed, initially with a sensitivity limit of about 0.5 ng/ml (Walker _et al_., 1973). Recent refinements of the procedure have resulted in a sensitivity limit of 0.05 ng/ml (Walker, to be published). At the outset of the isolation, a known quantity of a mixture of di-deutero and proteo DMT or alternatively di-deutero DMT alone is added to the sample, serving as an internal standard and carrier. A partially purified DMT fraction is obtained by a solvent extraction procedure and converted to a trimethylsilyl derivative. Final purification of the isolate and determination of the isotopic ratios is carried out with an LKB-9000 gas chromatograph mass spectrometer. Two pairs of ions are used for the isotopic ratio determination - the molecular ion signals at m/e 260 and 262 and the signals from the major fragmentation ion (the indole ring fragment) at m/e 202 and 204. Any change from the original isotopic ratio of the carrier can be related directly to the amount of endogenous DMT present in the sample.

Analysis of whole blood, plasma or serum for DMT revealed its presence (0.2-10 ng/ml) in 4 of 84 normal subjects, 6 of 35 acute schizophrenics, 4 of 46 chronic schizophrenics and 3 of 66 patients with other psychotic disorders. Some of these results have been reported by Lipinski _et al_. (1973), Wyatt _et al_. (1973a), and Bidder _et al_. (1974). The data indicate no marked differences among the groups, and no evidence has been found for the presence of DMT at concentrations approaching 40 ng/ml reported by Franzen and Gross (1965) or the submicrogram quantities suggested by the reports of Narasimhachari _et al_. (1971b). DMT was found in the urine at 0.1-1 ng/ml in 7 of 57 samples from patients with various psychoses (Bidder _et al_., 1974).

The infrequent occurrence of measurable DMT in blood and urine of patients with mental illness requires that a number of factors be considered as these results are not in accord with the DMT hypothesis. It is possible that the assay may not have sufficient sensitivity to differentiate between psychotic patients and normals. Peripheral levels may not reflect DMT concentrations in important tissues such as brain. Transient elevation in DMT may occur which can be seen only with frequent sampling of the same patient.

Finally, DMT may undergo very rapid metabolism in man.

To test the latter possibilities, experiments have been carried out wherein psychoactive doses (0.7 mg/kg) of DMT were administered i.m. to 11 normal subjects (Kaplan, 1974; Wyatt, 1974). Blood and urine levels of DMT were measured at various times and subjective symptoms were monitored. Blood DMT and the subjective "high" appeared to follow a similar time course. The absolute amounts of DMT found in blood and urine were quite small, despite the extremely intense behavioral effects. Not more than 2% of the injected dose of DMT could be recovered in blood and less than 0.2% was recovered in the urine. Thus, if a small amount of endogenous DMT were to be produced *in vivo*, it should not be surprising if this were not detectable in blood or urine, even if fortuitously the peak time chosen for obtaining the specimens. These experiments may explain why it was not possible to demonstrate marked differences in DMT levels between patients and normals. While the results of the analytical studies do not support the hypothesis that DMT is an endogenous psychotogen, they may explain why failure to find differences should not eliminate its further consideration.

In summary, these studies have demonstrated the presence of an enzyme in animal and human tissues which can form DMT *in vitro*. The biosynthesis of DMT was shown to occur in the rabbit *in vivo* and DMT was found to be rapidly metabolized in laboratory animals.

A sensitive and specific isotope dilution assay for the determination of DMT in body fluids was developed but it was not possible to confirm in a quantitative way the occurrence of elevated DMT in schizophrenia. Evidence was presented demonstrating that DMT is rapidly metabolized in man.

DMT fulfills some of the criteria required for its consideration as an endogenous substance of importance in schizophrenia. The most significant piece of negative evidence is the failure to find elevated DMT in blood in the majority of psychotic patients evaluated. On the other hand, DMT in single doses produces some schizophrenic-like symptoms, and enzymes for its synthesis are present in man. Tolerance does not develop upon repeated administration in some laboratory animals. Thus, DMT remains a candidate for playing a role at least in some types of schizophrenias.

Acknowledgements

The author acknowledges the collaboration of Dr. W.J.A. VandenHeuvel, Dr. H.S. Ahn and Mr. R.W. Walker of the Merck

Sharp & Dohme Research Laboratories for the development of the analytical procedures, Dr. R.J. Wyatt, J. Kaplan, and J.C. Gillin at the NIMH and St. Elizabeth's Hospital for participation in various phases of this study, Dr. T.G. Bidder of Case Western Reserve University, Dr. J. Lipinski of the Massachusetts General Hospital and Dr. E.F. Domino of the University of Michigan for the careful selection of clinical specimens for DMT measurements.

REFERENCES

Ahn, H.S., Walker, R.W., VandenHeuvel, W.J.A., Rosegay, A. and Mandel, L.R.: Studies on the in vivo biosynthesis of N,N-dimethyltryptamine (DMT) in the rabbit and rat. Fed. Proc. 32: 511, 1973.

Axelrod, J.: The enzymatic N-methylation of serotonin and other amines. J. Pharmacol. Exp. Ther. 138: 28-33, 1961.

Banarjee, S.P. and Snyder, S.H.: Methyltetrahydrofolic acid mediates N- and O-methylation of biogenic amines. Science 182: 74-75, 1973.

Bidder, T.G., Mandel, L.R., Ahn, H.S., Walker, R.W. and VandenHeuvel, W.J.A.: Blood and urinary DMT concentrations in acute psychotic disorders, Lancet 1: 165, 1974.

Cohen, I. and Vogel, W.H.: Determination and physiological disposition of dimethyltryptamine and diethyltryptamine in rat brain, liver, and plasma. Biochem. Pharmacol. 21: 1214-1218, 1972.

Franzen, Fr. and Gross, H.: Tryptamine, N,N-dimethyltryptamine, N,N-dimethyl-5-hydroxytryptamine and 5-methoxytryptamine in human blood and urine. Nature 206: 1052, 1965.

Greenberg, R.: N,N-dimethylated and N,N-diethylated indoleamines in schizophrenia. In Chemical Modulation of Brain Function,- A Tribute to J.E.P. Tolman, ed. by H.C. Sabelli, pp. 277-296, Raven Press, New York, 1973.

Gross, V.H. and Franzen, Fr.: Zur Bestimmung Koipereigener Amine in Biologischen Substraten. Zeitschrift Fur Klinische Chemie 3: 99-102, 1965.

Heller, B.: N-methylating enzyme in blood of schizophrenics. Psychosomatics 12: 273-274, 1971.

Himwich, H.E.: Indoleamines and the schizophrenias. In Biochemistry, Schizophrenias and Affective Illnesses, ed. by H.E. Himwich, pp. 79-112, Williams and Wilkins Co., Baltimore, 1971.

Hsu, L.L. and Mandell, A.J.: Multiple N-methyltransferase for aromatic alkylamines in brain. Life Sci. 13: 847-858, 1973.

Kaplan, J., Mandel, L.R., Walker, R.W., VandenHeuvel, W.J.A., Stillman, R., Gillin, J.C. and Wyatt, R.J.: Blood and urine levels of N,N-dimethyltryptamine following administration of psychoactive dosages to human subjects. Psychopharmacologia 38: 239, 1974.

Kety, S.S.: Current biochemical approaches to schizophrenia. New Engl. J. Med. 276: 325-331, 1967.

Lipinski, J., Mandel, L.R., Ahn, H.S., VandenHeuvel, W.J.A. and Walker, R.W.: Blood dimethyltryptamine concentrations in psychotic disorders. Biol. Psych. 9: 89, 1974.

Mandel, L.R., Rosenzweig, S. and Kuehl, F.A., Jr.: Purification and properties of indoleamine-N-methyltransferase. Biochem. Pharmacol. 20: 712-716, 1971.

Mandel, L.R., Ahn, H.S., VandenHeuvel, W.J.A. and Walker, R.W.: Indoleamine-N-methyltransferase in human lung. Biochem. Pharmacol. 21: 1197-1200, 1972.

Mandel, L.R., Rosegay, A., Walker, R.W., VandenHeuvel, W.J.A. and Rokach, J.: 5-Methyltetrahydrofolic acid as a mediator in the formation of pyridoindoles. Science 186: 741-743, 1974.

Mandell, A.J. and Morgan, M.: Indole(ethyl)amine N-methyltransferase in human brain. Nature 230: 85-87, 1971.

Morgan, M. and Mandell, A.J.: Indole(ethyl)amine N-methyltransferase in the brain. Science 165: 492-493, 1969.

Murphy, D.L. and Wyatt, R.J.: Reduced monoamine oxidase activity in blood platelets from schizophrenic patients. Nature 238: 225-226, 1972.

Narasimhachari, N., Heller, B., Spaide, J., Haskovec, L., Fugimori, M., Tabushi, K. and Himwich, H.E.: Urinary studies of schizophrenics and controls. Biol. Psychiat. 3: 9-20, 1971a.

Narasimhachari, N., Heller, B., Spaide, J., Haskovec, L., Meltzer, H., Strahilevitz, M. and Himwich, H.E.: N,N-Dimethylated indoleamines in blood. Biol. Psychiat. 3: 21-23, 1971b.

Narasimhachari, N., Plaut, J.M. and Himwich, H.E.: Indoleethylamine-N-methyltransferase in serum samples of schizophrenics and normal controls. Life Sci. 11: 221-227, 1972.

Rosengarten, H., Szemis, A., Piotrowski, A., Romaszewska, K., Matsumato, H., Stencka, K. and Jus, A.: N,N-Dimethyltryptamine and bufotenin in the urine of patients with chronic and acute schizophrenic psychoses. Psychiatria Polska 4: 519-521, 1970.

Saavedra, J.M. and Axelrod, J.: Psychotomimetic N-methylated tryptamines: Formation in brain _in vivo_ and _in vitro_. Science 172: 1365-1366, 1972.

Saavedra, J., Coyle, J.T. and Axelrod, J.: The distribution and properties of the nonspecific N-methyltransferase in brain. J. Neurochem. 20: 743-752, 1973.

Shulgin, A.T.: Some qualitative properties of the psychotomimetics. Neurosciences Res. Prog. Bull. 8: 72-78, 1970.

Szára, S.: Hallucinogenic amines and schizophrenia. In Amines and Schizophrenia, ed. by H.E. Himwich, S.S. Kety, and J.R. Smythies, pp. 181-197, Pergamon Press, 1967.

Thithapandha, A.: Substrate specificity and heterogeneity of N-methyltransferase. Biochem. Biophys. Res. Comm. 47: 301-308, 1972.

Walker, R.W., Ahn, H.S., Mandel, L.R. and VandenHeuvel, W.J.A.: Identification of N,N-dimethyltryptamine as the product of an _in vitro_ enzymatic methylation. Anal. Biochem. 47: 228-234, 1972.

Walker, R.W., Ahn, H.S., Albers-Schonberg, G., Mandel, L.R. and VandenHeuvel, W.J.A.: Gas chromatographic-mass spectrometric isotope dilution assay for N,N-dimethyltryptamine in human plasma. Biochem. Med. 8: 105-113, 1973.

Wyatt, R.J., Gillin, J.C., Kaplan, J., Stillman, R., Mandel, L.R., Ahn, H.S., VandenHeuvel, W.J.A. and Walker, R.W.: N,N-Dimethyltryptamine - A possible relationship to schizophrenia. In Serotonin-New Vistas, Advances in Biochemical Psychopharmacology, Vol. 11, ed. by E. Costa, pp. 299-313, Raven Press, New York, 1974.

Wyatt, R.J., Mandel, L.R., Ahn, H.S., Walker, R.W. and VandenHeuvel, W.J.A.: Gas chromatographic-mass spectrometric isotope dilution determination of N,N-dimethyltryptamine concentrations in normals and pyschiatric patients. Psychopharmacologia 31: 265-270, 1973a.

Wyatt, R.J., Murphy, D.L., Belmaker, R., Donelly, C., Cohen, S. and Pollin, W.: Reduced monoamine oxidase activity in platelets: A possible genetic marker for vulnerability to schizophrenia. Science 179: 916-918, 1973b.

Wyatt, R.J., Saavedra, J.M. and Axelrod, J.: A dimethyltryptamine (DMT) forming enzyme in human blood. Amer. J. Psychiat. 130: 754-760, 1973c.

Neurotransmitter Balances Regulating Behavior,
edited and published by E.F. Domino and
J.M. Davis, Ann Arbor, © 1975

INDOLE ALKYL AMINES AS PSYCHOTOGEN PRECURSORS -- POSSIBLE NEUROTRANSMITTER IMBALANCE

Edward F. Domino
Department of Pharmacology
University of Michigan
Ann Arbor, Michigan
and Lafayette Clinic
Detroit, Michigan

One of the concerns of a pharmacologist is to develop new therapeutic drugs. An area of great need is to obtain better drugs to treat schizophrenic patients. How does one develop new drugs? The answer is to use animal models of human disease. Currently there are a number of drug models of psychoses which have been proposed including LSD-25 and related agents, drugs blocking cholinergic function, phencyclidine, chronic amphetamine, and cannabis intoxication (Cole _et al_., 1973). The amphetamine model is by far the best known and extensively utilized in screening for new antipsychotic drugs. It is well known that chronic amphetamine dependence leads to a paranoid schizophrenia-like state that sometimes is very difficult to distinguish from endogenous psychosis (Connell, 1958; Ellinwood, 1969). This model is especially suitable to study in animals (Randrup _et al_., 1963; Ellinwood and Sudilovsky, 1973). In low doses amphetamine produces an alerting response and an increase in motor activity. Still larger doses produce behavioral stereotypes. Current neuroleptic drugs are very effective in antagonizing either the locomotor and/or stereotyped behavior. Snyder (1972) has suggested that _d_-amphetamine acts mainly through a norepinephrine (NE) mechanism that produces increased psychomotor activity, while _l_-amphetamine acts through a dopamine (DA) mechanism that produces stereotyped behavior. Neuroleptics such as chlorpromazine, which antagonize both NE and DA, shift the dose-effect curve of _d_-amphetamine to the right for both locomotor activity and stereotypes. On the other hand, more selective DA antagonists like haloperidol antagonize mainly the stereotypes. Many extremely useful antipsychotic drugs for the management of schizophrenic patients have been developed from the amphetamine psychosis model. There is no doubt that the amphetamine model is one of the best in producing a neuropsychiatric disturbance in a previously normal animal. We need to thank our colleagues in the pharmaceutical industry for properly exploiting the amphetamine animal model.

Current antipsychotic drugs, found on the basis of the amphetamine model, are useful in treating about two of every three schizophrenic patients. I would like to focus on the one of three patients resistant to current antipsychotic drugs inasmuch as these are the ones with the greatest need for newer types of medication. My interest has shifted toward the indole hallucinogens. Our current antipsychotic drugs such as chlorpromazine and haloperidol are very poor antagonists of LSD-25 and DMT. It is now widely recognized that such neuroleptics are of little value and may actually make some patients on a bad LSD-25 trip worse. In fact, talking the patient on LSD-25 "down" is a much better therapeutic approach. It seems reasonable to look for selective antagonists of indole hallucinogens which can be made endogenously as another model of psychosis to examine extensively. I have been encouraged by Dr. Gottlieb of the Lafayette Clinic to pursue this approach.

The literature on indole hallucinogens and schizophrenia is rather confusing. This is because investigators who have access to schizophrenic patients do not have sophisticated gas chromatographic-mass spectrographic (GC-MS) facilities, and those chemically sophisticated researchers who have such analytic facilities do not have access to a suitable patient research population. This situation has existed for some time and probably will continue to exist for a long time to come. The current nature of psychiatric research strategy, funding, social and legal pressures regarding informed consent and commitment of the mentally ill (Szasz, 1974) all combine to retard progress. This situation has become so confusing in Michigan in the last few years that most research with mental patients has stopped. In attempting to protect the rights of the mentally ill, their rights to proper diagnoses and better treatments are being discarded.

The interested reader can find a large literature in which various fluorescent, paper, thin layer and/or gas chromatographic techniques have been utilized to determine the presence of hallucinogenic indoles such as tryptamine (T), dimethyltryptamine (DMT) and 5-hydroxydimethyltryptamine (bufotenin, BFT) in various body fluids. Almost all investigators agree that very small amounts of such indoles, if any, are present in human fluids. Inasmuch as most chemical methods have borderline sensitivity in detecting picogram amounts of such compounds, it is little wonder that the literature on this subject is chaotic. Emphasis must be placed on the reliability of the methods used in any particular study. Much of the older literature on the presence of hallucinogenic indoles in the blood and urine of schizophrenic patients with and without administration of L-methionine, L-tryptophan (TP) and/or MAO inhibitors is described in books by Himwich et al. (1967), Himwich (1971), Weil-Malherbe and Szara (1971) and reviews by Domino (1969), Kety (1967) and Wyatt et al. (1971). Rather than go over what has already been thoroughly reviewed of this older literature, I would like to concentrate on five critical questions and offer evidence, pro or con, that bears on them.

I. Can known hallucinogenic indoles be made biosynthetically in living organisms, especially in man? Figure 1 summarizes some of the biosynthetic pathways proposed in the formation of known hallucinogenic indoles. Their ultimate source is the essential amino acid TP. An individual's diet is the major source of TP, although it can be made biosynthetically via chorismate and several intermediates to indole-3-glycerolphosphate and thence to TP (Dagley and Nicholson, 1970). The metabolism of TP is complex (Guroff and Lovenberg, 1970; Fernstrom and Wurtman, 1974). Most of the TP is utilized by cells to form essential proteins. About 1% of the TP is hydroxylated to form 5-hydroxytryptophan (5-HTP). Another portion is converted in the liver by tryptophan oxygenase (L-tryptophan: oxygen oxidoreductase, tryptophan pyrrolase) to form kynurenine (KYN), quinolate and thence nicotinate, the essential vitamin B_3 necessary to form the cofactors nicotinamide adenine dinucleotide (NAD) and nicotinamide adenine dinucleotide phosphate (NADP). A very small portion of TP is decarboxylated by aromatic amino acid decarboxylase (AAAD) to T. The same enzyme also decarboxylates 5-HTP to 5-hydroxytryptamine (5-HT, serotonin).

There is evidence that T (Martin and Sloan, 1970), BFT (Fabing and Hawkins, 1956; Fabing, 1956; Fisher, 1968) and DMT (Szara, 1956, 1957) are hallucinogenic in man. These same substances are constituents of various snuffs taken by certain South American Indian tribes. The evidence, pro and con, that some of these compounds are hallucinogenic as well as proof that they are constituents of various snuffs has been elegantly summarized by Holmstedt and Lindgren (1967). These substances have significant autonomic and motor effects. There is some question as to whether BFT is hallucinogenic (Isbell, 1967). Studies in animals indicate that 5-methoxy DMT (5-MeODMT is more behaviorally toxic than DMT (Gessner and Page, 1962; Benington et al., 1965; Vasko et al., 1974). Hence, 5-MeODMT is of special significance. Shulgin (1974) has data that

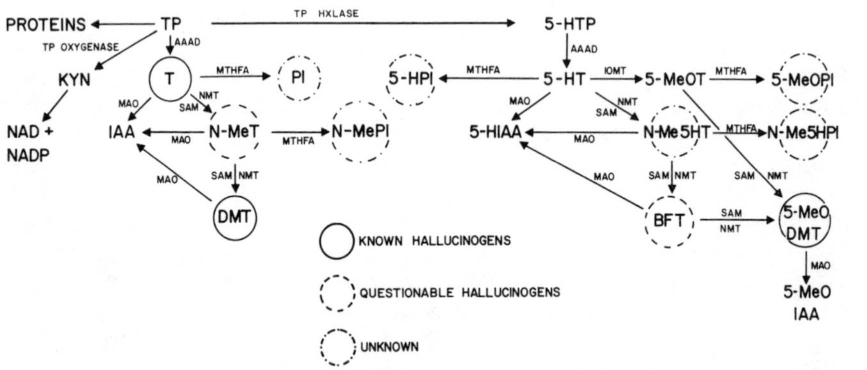

Fig. 1. Possible formation of hallucinogenic amines from tryptophan. TP, an essential amino acid, is derived primarily from the diet. Most of it is converted to proteins. Via TP oxygenase, it is biotransformed to KYN and ultimately to the essential cofactors NAD and NADP. About 1% of TP is converted via TP hydroxylase (TP HXLASE) to 5-HTP. AAAD converts both TP and 5-HT to T and especially 5-HT. Normally, type A and B MAO biotransform T to the corresponding aldehyde. Aldehyde dehydrogenase converts it to indoleacetic acid (IAA). Type A MAO biotransforms 5-HT and in a similar manner 5-hydroxyindoleacetic acid (5-HIAA) is formed. NMT also can convert T to DMT and 5-HT to BFT. These tertiary amines are poorer substrates for MAO than their corresponding primary amines. Nevertheless, they are converted to IAA and 5-HIAA. Indole-O-methyltransferase (IOMT) can also convert 5-HT to 5-MeODMT. MAO oxidizes 5-MeOT and ultimately 5-MeOIAA. The known hallucinogens, T, DMT, and 5-MeODMT, are enclosed in solid circles. The questionable hallucingens are enclosed with interrupted circles. They include BFT and many pyridoindoles (PI).

5-MeODMT is a potent hallucinogen in man. The intoxication produced is qualitatively like DMT but 5-MeODMT is more potent. The effective dose is 10 mg, and usually less. The onset of action is within one minute and is shorter in duration than DMT. Both hallucinogens are ineffective orally and must be given parenterally. The inhalation route is usually employed. The N-homologs (N,N-diethyl and N,N-diisopropyl-5-methoxytryptamine) are less potent as is true of their counterparts without the 5-methoxy group. Again, all of these agents must be given parenterally to be effective.

It is a paradox that nature should provide us with the biosynthetic pathways for making hallucinogenic indoles. Axelrod (1962) first reported the presence of a nonspecific N-methyl transferase (NMT) in rabbit lung capable of forming N-methyltryptamine (NMET) from T and S-adenosylmethionine (SAM), and DMT from NMET and SAM. This reaction is summarized in figure 2. If ^{14}C-SAM is used, one can easily measure labeled indole products. However, other substances can also be methylated so great care must be taken to prove the labelled product is indeed ^{14}C-DMT. Both Mandel (1975) and ourselves have shown, by TLC separations, that T is converted primarily to NMET. When NMET is used, it is readily converted to DMT by the rabbit lung enzyme. Amazingly, Axelrod's important observation was not pursued for about seven years. Then other investigators observed a similar enzyme as well as a more specific indole amine-N-methyl transferase (INMT) in many tissues of both animals (Morgan and Mandell, 1969; Mandel et al., 1971; Saavedra and Axelrod, 1972a; Thithapandha, 1972; Walker et al., 1972; Ahn et al., 1973; Hsu and Mandell, 1973; Saavedra et al., 1973) and man (Heller, 1971; Mandell and Morgan, 1971; Mandel et al., 1972; Narasimhachari et al., 1972; Wyatt et al., 1973c; Domino et al., 1973).

In addition to SAM, 5-methyltetrahydrofolic acid (MTHF) has been reported to be an alternative methyl donor for forming DMT (Banerjee and Snyder, 1973; Hsu and Mandell, 1973). However, Mandel (1974) has been unable to show that it acts as a methyl donor for NMT. Mandel et al. (1974) have obtained evidence that MTHF can contribute a methyl group to T to form a tricyclic norharmaline alkaloid which they called a pyridoindole. Presumably, a formaldehyde forming enzyme is involved. Barchas et al. (1974) have shown that a similar substance, which they called tryptoline, is formed from T and MTHF by human platelets. In addition, the same group (Wyatt et al., 1975a) have also shown that the human brain contains a similar enzyme to form tryptoline from T and a large series of related

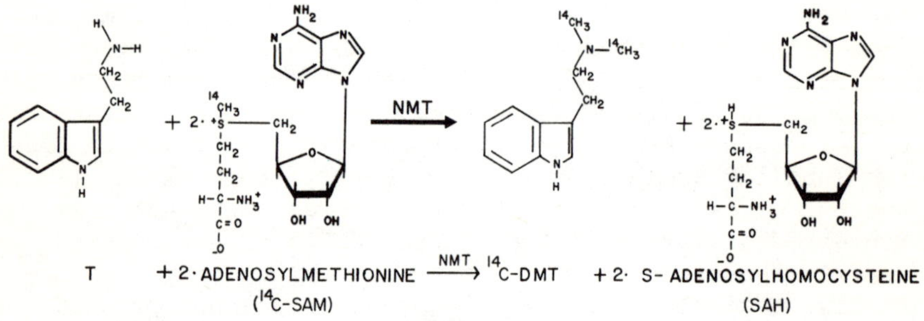

Fig. 2. Synthesis of ^{14}C-DMT by N-methyltransferase using ^{14}C-SAM. The overall reaction of T and two molecules of ^{14}C-SAM is shown to form ^{14}C-DMT and two molecules of SAH. There is some disagreement among investigators based upon the Km's of both T and NMET as to how easily T can form DMT. In our laboratory we can easily demonstrate that DMT was formed from NMET. Using T as the substrate, we found only NMET under our in vitro conditions.

tryptoline derivatives from other indole alkylamine substrates. This class of compounds has also been called 1,2,3,4-tetrahydro-β-carbolines, 9H-1,2,3,4,-tetrahydropyrido(3,4-6)indoles, and 1,2,3,4-tetrahydronorharmans. Their formation is illustrated in figure 3. For priority purposes, it should be pointed out that such compounds were first suggested by McIsaac (1961a) to be produced from 5-HT in schizophrenic patients. McIsaac (1961b) obtained some evidence that the urine of rats given 5-methoxy T, ethanol or acetaldehyde, iproniazid and disulfiram contained 1-methyl-6-methoxy-1,2,3,4-tetrahydro-2-carboline. The very

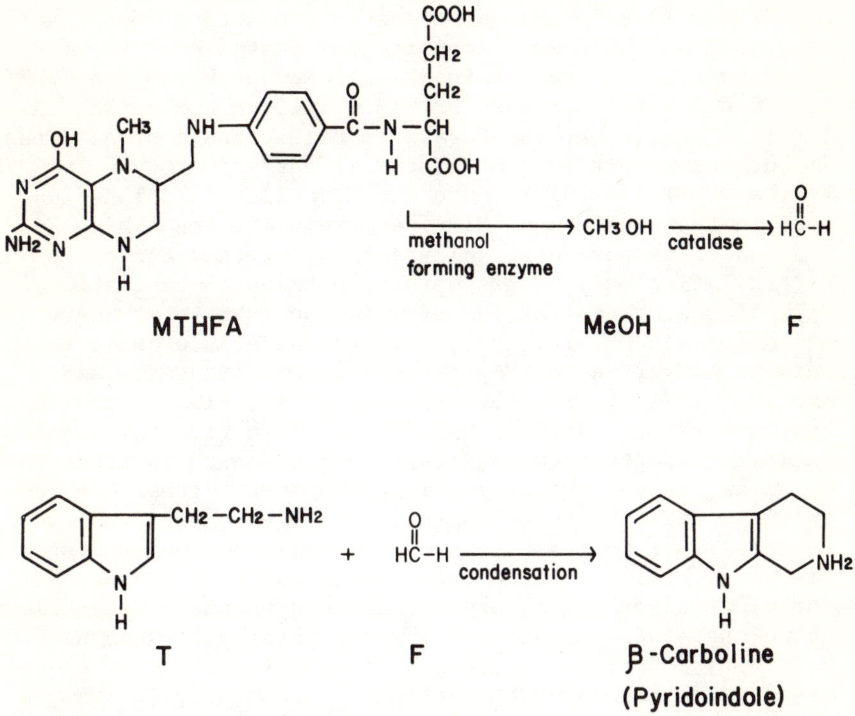

Fig. 3. Possible formation of pyridoindoles from 5-methyltetrahydrofolic acid and tryptamine. As yet, it is not clear if MTHF donates a methyl group to form methanol which is subsequently converted to formaldehyde and then condensation with tryptamine (T) to form a pyridoloindole or an enzyme exists that directly incorporates a methyl group from MTHF into the pyridoindole.

recent findings of Mandel et al. (1974), Barchas et al., (1974) and Wyatt et al. (1975a) are a potent stimulus for further research into the pharmacology of all β-carbolines including the naturally occurring alkaloids harmine and harmaline which have long been known to be hallucinogenic. Lin and Narasimhachari (1974) have been unable to show that MTHF is involved in the O-methylation or N-methylation of 5-HT. Rather, they suggest the indole-N may be methylated. Hence, the role of MTHF in the precise methylation of indoles is still controversial.

Mandel et al. (1971) reported that INMT from rabbit lung

had a Km for T of $3.3x10^{-4}$M and for NMET of $5x10^{-5}$M. Mandel et al. (1972) reported that with the purified human lung enzyme NMET had the lowest Km of several indole amine substrates ($2.8x10^{-4}$M) and that the products of the reaction, BFT and DMT, were inhibitory. Saavedra et al. (1973) reported that for rat brain NMT the Km for both T and NMET is 2.8 and $3.7x10^{-5}$M and for SAM $5.1x10^{-5}$M. Research in our laboratories at the Lafayette Clinic has indicated that Km for the rabbit lung NMT for T is approximately $7.7x10^{-4}$M and for NMET $1.5x10^{-4}$M. Hsu and Mandell have pointed out that in the presence of MTHF rat brain NMT has a high Km and hence low enzyme affinity indicating that enzymatic N-methylation only occurs with high amine concentrations. High tissue concentrations of T in the rabbit, at least, are made into DMT in vivo. T given intracisternally to rats is converted to NMET as well as DMT (Saavedra and Axelrod, 1972a). Furthermore, Ahn et al. (1973) have shown that the rabbit can make DMT from NMET in vivo. It is especially important to note that most researchers agree that in human tissues the enzymatic activity of either the non-specific NMT or the more specific INMT enzyme is very low, especially if the samples are not dialyzed. Our own studies using brain tissue obtained from autopsy of deceased chronic schizophrenic, organic brain syndrome or mentally normal patients who died of various physical causes have been very sobering. We have been able to find only extremely low levels of NMT activity in human brain. Furthermore, we have been unable to find a difference in regional NMT activity among those three groups of patients in brain samples not subjected to dialysis (Domino et al., 1973). Narasimhachari et al. (1972) reported enhanced NMT activity in the serum of most acute and some chronic schizophrenic patients. Wyatt et al. (1973c) have also reported enhanced NMT activity in the platelets of schizophrenic patients compared to mentally normal controls. When the enzyme from both the normal controls and the schizophrenic patients was dialyzed, it showed similar activity, suggesting that the schizophrenic platelets lacked a small dialyzable inhibitor. Demethylated SAM, better known as S-adenosyl-homocysteine (SAH), immediately comes to mind as a possibility inasmuch as this agent is a potent NMT inhibitor as discussed below.

It is well known that the amine substrates for forming the methylated indoles exist in various tissues of animals and man. These include 5-HT (Lewis, 1958; Garattini and Valzelli, 1965) and T (Martin et al., 1972; Saavedra and Axelrod, 1972b; Sloan et al., 1974). In addition, living organisms contain adequate levels of the N-methyl donors

SAM (Baldessarini and Kopin, 1966; Gaitonde, 1970) and the MTHF (Korevaar *et al.*, 1973). After the MAO inhibitor isocarboxazid, dog brain and spinal cord T is increased 2-3 fold (Martin *et al.*, 1972). Both isocarboxazid and pargyline increase dog blood T as well, but isocarboxazid does not elevate cat brain T levels (Sloan *et al.*, 1974). Frohman (1973) and Gottlieb and Frohman (1974) have suggested that these biosynthetic pathways for forming hallucinogenic indoles are excessively utilized in schizophrenic patients with a plasma alpha helical S protein. According to their view, this protein facilitates the uptake of TP into cells and makes TP more available for all of the synthetic pathways shown in figure 1.

Conclusion. It seems fairly certain that the biosynthetic pathways for making hallucinogenic indoles exist in many tissues in animals and man. The non-specific NMT enzyme has a rather high Km for substrates such as T and NMET indicating that rather high tissue levels need to be present in order for DMT to be formed. Furthermore, in man the NMT and INMT enzymes have rather low levels of activity. Hence, although the biosynthetic pathways for the formation of indole hallucinogens exist, these pathways probably are not very active unless the patient has high levels of substrate in tissues containing these enzymes or lacks endogenous NMT inhibitors. The enhanced platelet NMT activity in schizophrenic patients is due to a decrease of a dialyzable endogenous inhibitor. The fact that SAH is a potent product inhibitor of this enzymatic reaction suggests that this and other endogenous substances (see below) should be measured in platelets of schizophrenic patients and compared with normals. The fact that MTHF can act as a methyl donor to form pyridoindoles *in vitro* suggests that a similar mechanism might occur *in vivo* which would lead to a whole new series of possible hallucinogens.

II. *Do hallucinogenic indoles really exist in the body fluids of schizophrenic patients in suffient concentrations to be psychotogenic?* Not long ago the answer to this question would have been a qualified "yes" (Franzen and Gross, 1965; Gross and Franzen, 1965; Fisher, 1968; Rosengarten *et al.*, 1970; Narasimhachari *et al.*, 1971a,b; Greenberg, 1973; Himwich *et al.*, 1973). Now the answer seems a qualified "no" - at least for the majority of schizophrenics because of the recent publications of Mandel (1974a) and his associates who used a GC-MS isotope dilution assay specific for DMT (Bidder *et al.*, 1974; Lipinski *et al.*, 1974; Walker *et al.*, 1973; Wyatt *et al.*, 1973a, 1974). Their studies indicate that a large percentage of acute and chronic schizophrenic patients have no significant plasma levels of DMT to the minimum detection level of their assay, which was 0.5-1.8 ng/ml of plasma. It was not stated why plasma instead of whole blood was used. Amines such as 5-HT are taken up by platelets, so the distribution of DMT in the blood elements is essential to examine. These researchers made a very sobering observation when they gave DMT in hallucinogenic doses to mentally normal volunteers (Kaplan et al., 1974a). They were only able to measure very small plasma levels of DMT for a very short time using the same GC-MS assay method, indicating that this hallucinogen disappears from the plasma very rapidly. This finding in man is in agreement with data in rats using a less specific fluorometric method (Cohen and Vogel, 1972). Narasimhachari et al. (1974) reported positive identification of both BFT and DMT in the urine of six drug free chronic schizophrenic patients placed on a diet low in foods containing preformed indoleamines. The patients showed exacerbation of their symptoms during the drug free period of 13 weeks in which urines were assayed after the 4th week of their drug holiday. BFT was identified for all six patients using TLC separation and confirmation by GC-MS. Very low urinary levels of DMT were also found using TLC separation and identification by GC-MS. The base peak at m/e 58 was used primarily for quantification. However, the mass spectra of the DMT standard and a DMT peak urine sample were identical. The fact that a small percentage of schizophrenic patients have detectable plasma or urine levels of DMT indicates that they probably produce endogenously very large amounts of this substance. Investigators who have used chromatographic assays have consistently reported enhanced blood or urine levels of DMT and related indoles (Narasimhachari et al., 1971a,b; Greenberg, 1973; Himwich et al., 1973). It would appear that these latter investigators were measuring not only DMT but also other amines with similar retention times. Hence, the issue of whether schizophrenic patients have enhanced hallucinogen levels is still wide open. It is especially important to measure T, BFT, DMT and 5-MODMT simultaneously before and during TP and methionine loading with and without an MAO inhibitor in both normals and schizophrenic patients of all types before this question can be answered definitively.

Conclusion. Investigators who have used nonspecific chemical assay methods for measuring DMT and related substances report enhanced levels in the blood or urine of schizophrenic patients. However, when a very specific isotope dilution GC-MS technique for DMT was used, the vast majority of schizophrenic patients did not have enhanced plasma DMT levels. Further studies are obviously indicated not only because other amines may be involved but also because of low plasma levels and very rapid disappearance of DMT given in hallucinogenic doses to mentally normal controls. Schizophrenic patients in whose blood DMT is detected obviously must synthesize enormous amounts endogenously. Those investigators who report DMT to be present in the blood of a large number of schizophrenics tend to use whole blood, while those who report it to be absent in the majority of patients use plasma or serum. Hence, the relative distribution of DMT in the blood elements needs to be studied further.

III. Does tolerance occur to DMT? Even if DMT were present in schizophrenic patients, it might be argued that tolerance might occur to this hallucinogen as with LSD-25. This argument was used previously that even if LSD-25 could be made biosynthetically it could not be an endogenous hallucinogen. However, the tolerance argument is not valid for cyclic tolerance to LSD-25 has been observed, at least in the goat (Koella et al., 1964). Cyclic tolerance might, in fact, explain why schizophrenic patients have remissions and exacerbations of their illness. Furthermore, schizophrenic patients might have disturbed tolerance mechanisms. Hence, the tolerance argument is not critical as to whether an endogenous hallucinogen is psychotogenic. Still, it is of interest to ask if DMT produces tolerance. Gillin et al. (1973) reported that tolerance to daily DMT does not occur in cats. Similarly, Kaplan et al. (1974b) were unable to show tolerance to DMT in squirrel monkeys, mice and human volunteers. DMT in a dose of 0.7 mg/kg i.m. twice daily for 5 consecutive days to 6 subjects did not produce tolerance even when the second injection of DMT followed the first by less than 3 hr. These investigators neglected a basic pharmacologic principle, emphasized by Seevers and Deneau (1963) that in order to produce tolerance to a substance one needs to maintain high blood and tissue levels of the chemical 24 hr a day for many weeks. Hence, we decided to reevaluate this problem using hungry albino Holtzman rats trained to bar press for a sugar-sweetened milk reward. When DMT was given in a dose of 10 mg/kg i.p. bar pressing behavior in the rat stopped for a short time in a dose related manner (Kovacic and Domino, 1973). When DMT was given every 2 hr for 21 days bar pressing behavior ceased for several days as though there was an initial sensitization. After several weeks tolerance to this phenomenon was observed. A small dose (0.1 mg/kg) of LSD-25 given to DMT tolerant animals also showed some cross-tolerance. Partial tolerance between LSD-25 and DMT was symmetric. Animals given LSD-25 daily became tolerant to this hallucinogen. When they were then given small doses of DMT disruption of bar pressing behavior was less than that observed in naive animals. However, large doses of DMT still disrupted bar pressing behavior in LSD-25 tolerant animals. It was concluded that tolerance occurs to the behavioral disruptive effects of DMT with partial cross-tolerance to LSD-25 (Kovacic and Domino, 1974). These findings are consistent with those of Rosenberg et al. (1964) in which DMT was given to human subjects highly tolerant to LSD-25. Rosenberg et al. pointed out that except for the shorter onset and duration of action the peak effects of DMT in doses of 0.5 mg/kg in non-tolerant humans were similar to those produced by 1.5 μg/kg of LSD-25. Subjects given LSD-25 twice daily to a maximum dose of 3.0 μg/kg showed marked tolerance. On the other hand, DMT, in an i.m. dose of 0.5 to 1.0 mg/kg, produced only a mild degree of cross-tolerance to the mental response. There was no cross-tolerance to the pupillary effects of DMT. The nature of Rosenberg et al.'s experimental design would have favored demonstration of a high degree of cross-tolerance between LSD-25 and DMT.

It is of interest that chronic schizophrenic patients usually do not respond to DMT (Szára, 1967) as much as do normal subjects. This has often been interpreted as due to the fact that schizophrenic patients are apathetic and do not verbalize their feelings as readily. However, there are psychotropic drugs schizophrenic patients tolerate very poorly. For example, it is well known that schizophrenic patients do not tolerate the psychotomimetic phencyclidine (Domino and Luby, 1973). Such patients are made considerably worse. Similarly, amphetamines and methylphenidate may activate some schizophrenic patients. Schizophrenic patients do not tolerate MAO inhibitors (Ban, 1969), particularly tranylcypromine, especially if combined with TP and/or methionine (Alexander et al., 1963; Sprintz et al., 1963). Schizophrenic patients also are very sensitive to the administration of the dopamine β-hydroxylase and alcohol dehydrogenase inhibitor, disulfiram (Antabuse), as reported by Heath et al. (1965). The fact that these latter drugs activate the schizophrenic process would suggest that the resistance of schizophrenics to DMT could be interpreted as partial tolerance to an endogenous psychotogenic substance. Tolerance to any psychoactive substance can be due to a) behavioral mechanisms, b) enhanced biotransformation or c) an unknown cellular adaptive process. It would be of great interest to determine the pharmacokinetics of indole hallucinogens, especially in their blood formed elements and plasma half-life as well as their possible differential biotransformation in normals and schizophrenic patients. Szára (1961) and his associates (Szára and Axelrod, 1959; Szára _et al._, 1962) suggested that the biological effects of N-dialkyltryptamines may be due to biotransformation to corresponding 6-hydroxy metabolites. Jaccarini and Jepson (1968) provided evidence that human liver tissue obtained at autopsy could effectively 6-hydroxylate tryptamine and DMT, but only weakly N-acetyltryptophan. However, liver microsomes obtained from a patient who died of a barbiturate overdose caused considerable hydroxylation of this latter substrate. These investigators pointed out that this is in keeping with their previous findings in rats and rabbits that phenobarbital is a potent inducer of indole-6-hydroxylase activity against indolic substrates which are normally poorly hydroxylated, but not against substrates that normally are well hydroxylated. However, Holmstedt and Lindgren (1967) could find no evidence of such a pathway of metabolism. Furthermore, Rosenberg _et al._ (1963) compared DMT and 6-hydroxy DMT given i.m. in doses up to 1 mg/kg to former opiate addicts who had no major signs of physical illness or psychosis. It was quite apparent from their study that DMT provoked a marked subjective response with objective physiological changes while a similar dose of 6-hydroxy DMT produced only minimal actions. Thus, in man the 6-hydroxy active metabolite hypothesis does not appear to be valid. It is generally known that hydroxyl substitutions produce compounds that penetrate the blood brain barrier poorly as, for example, 5-HT and BFT in contrast to T and DMT. Nevertheless, additional research on the biotransformation of indole hallucinogens in a large variety of animals and man and comparative metabolic studies in mentally normal and schizophrenic patients is essential to develop new treatment approaches as discussed below.

Conclusion. Tolerance to DMT does occur especially with high and frequent doses given for a prolonged period. It does not occur with relatively infrequent doses. However, this does not rule out a possible psychotogenic role of this agent in schizophrenia. Additional pharmacokinetic and metabolic studies of DMT and related hallucinogens in animals and man are essential.

IV. What are effective approaches for preventing the synthesis, enhancing the breakdown or antagonizing the effects of hallucinogenic indoles? Some of the possible therapeutic approaches to treating those schizophrenic patients who produce hallucinogenic indoles are summarized in table 1. Inasmuch as TP is an essential amino acid that humans cannot biosynthesize in sufficient quantity, one

Table 1

Possible Therapeutic Approaches to Treating Patients Producing An Excess of Indole Hallucinogens

1. Low TP diet + nicotinamide.
2. Selective competitors with TP for AAAD.
3. Enhance TP oxygenase activity.
4. Selective inhibitors of NMT and INMT.
5. Compounds which trap methyl groups from SAM and MTHF, penetrate BBB, and are pharmacologically inactive.
6. Enhance breakdown of indole hallucinogens.
    a. MAO
    b. Demethylation
    c. N-oxide formation
    d. Hydroxylation (?)
7. Indole hallucinogen antagonists
    a. Methiothepin (?)

approach could be to reduce TP intake in selected patients. One of the major problems is to reduce the TP content of the diet to a sufficient degree that would still be palatable and sufficiently nutritious to maintain life. Himwich (1971) used this approach in the treatment of a few schizophrenic patients. Unfortunately, his low TP diet did not improve the patients. However, no blood TP measurements were done in order to determine how effective the diet was. In addition, one would have to select schizophrenic patients on the basis that they produce excessive hallucinogenic indoles, otherwise a low TP diet would be of little value. The low TP diet seems an especially rational approach in view of its analogy to the low phenylalanine diet in the treatment of phenylketonuric children. Of course, nicotinic acid supplements would have to be given to patients on a low TP diet to prevent pellagra. It is of interest that many schizophrenic patients eat very poorly during an exacerbation of their illness. Whether this makes the mental disturbance worse or is beneficial to the patient is not known. It is a fact that acute schizophrenics have plasma TP levels significantly below normal (Gilmour et al., 1973; Manowitz et al., 1973; Domino and Krause, 1974a). As the acute patients recover in the hospital, plasma TP levels gradually return toward normal. Manowitz et al. and Gilmour et al. pointed out that acute schizophrenic patients had normal plasma phenylalanine and tyrosine levels at a time when plasma TP was reduced. They concluded that the selective decrease in TP could not be due to starvation but they did not do a food deprivation control to rule this out. It is well known that during periods of starvation and stress, such as prisoners held in concentration camps or patients undergoing severe weight reducing diets, there is an increased incidence of psychoses. Mentally normal people with severe dietary restrictions in the face of great stress would presumably have low plasma TP levels but in addition probably low levels of many other important nutrients as well. Our present knowledge does not allow one to make a definitive conclusion as to whether selective low TP intake in schizophrenic patients would be beneficial. Obviously, such a therapeutic approach would be relatively simple and could surely be justified on grounds of its potential merit. However, one must be certain that the patient is an indole hallucinogen producer and that blood TP measurements be taken to insure proper low TP intake.

As previously discussed, four major enzymes are involved in the biosynthesis of hallucinogenic indoles (see figure 1). Aromatic amino acid decarboxylase (AAAD) is responsible for the decarboxylation of TP to T. Normally, very low levels of brain T are present and after a MAO inhibitor the levels of T increase 2-3 fold but there are marked species differences as mentioned earlier (Martin et al., 1972; Sloan et al., 1974). AAAD is also involved in the decarboxylation of 5-HTP to 5-HT. There are much higher levels of 5-HT than T in the brain; apparently 5-HTP is a much more effective substrate than TP for AAAD. The use of synthetic TP derivatives such as α-methyltryptophan would be an interesting approach to reduce brain levels of T and 5-HT. The rationale would be analogous to that of α-methyl DOPA as a competing substrate for L-DOPA. α-Methyltryptophan has been shown to cause a prolonged decrease in brain 5-HT (Sourkes, 1971). A similar reduction in brain T would be expected. This agent also induces TP oxygenase activity in the liver which would further shunt TP away from the synthesis of hallucinogenic indoles. Selective 5-HTP supplements might be necessary to maintain brain 5-HT at reasonable levels. One of the disadvantages of α-methyltryptophan is that probably α-methyltryptamine would accumulate as a false neurotransmitter. Inasmuch as α-methyltryptamine is psychotoxic in both man (Murphree *et al.*, 1961) and animals (Vasko *et al.*, 1974), the limiting factor to this therapeutic approach would be its accumulation in the brain.

Since T and 5-HT are substrates of both a nonspecific NMT and a more specific INMT, another approach would be to find selective inhibitors of these enzymes. An important clue is the fact that SAH and DMT are product inhibitors of the NMT from rabbit lung (Krause and Domino, 1974). As shown in figure 4, SAH is an especially potent inhibitor of the rabbit lung enzyme as was first shown by a medical student, Ms. Bonnie Smith, and a premedical student, Mr. Laurence Domino, working in my laboratory at the University of Michigan in the summer of 1972. Since then, Lin *et al.* (1973) have described further the kinetics of SAH inhibition. It is known that SAH also inhibits a wide variety of methyltransferase reactions including phenethanolamine N-methyltransferase (PNMT) which catalyzes the methylation of norepinephrine to epinephrine (Deguchi and Barchas, 1972), catechol-O-methyltransferase (COMT) which methylates norepinephrine to normetanephrine (Deguchi and Barchas, 1972; Coward *et al.*, 1972), indole O-methyltransferase (IOMT), which forms melatonin from acetylserotonin (Deguchi and Barchas, 1972), nicotinamide N-methyltransferase which forms N-methylnicotinamide (Swiatek *et al.*, 1973), SAM-homocysteine-S-methyl transferase which forms methionine (Shapiro *et al.*, 1965), glycine methyl-transferase which forms sarcosine (Kerr, 1972), histamine N-methyltransferase which forms N-methylhistamine (Zappia *et al.*, 1969), and tRNA methyltransferase which forms methylated polynucleotides (Kerr, 1972). Methylation of DNA which involves SAM as the methyl donor has been suggested as playing a role in switching off genes when their need in development is over (Adams, 1973). SAH should be studied as an inhibitor of this methylation reaction.

In view of the lack of specificity of SAH as a methyltransferase inhibitor *in vitro*, it probably is fairly toxic *in vivo*. However, I do not know of any data on the pharmacology and toxicology of SAH. There would be no great harm to the patient if PNMT and COMT were inhibited. Inhibition of IOMT would reduce melatonin levels which would not be too crucial for man and would be beneficial because 5-MeODMT would not be formed. Since methionine is already in the diet, its formation *in vivo* from homocysteine does not seem important nor does the N-methylation of histamine. The only systems which might be adversely affected by inhibition are the methylation of tRNA and DNA, but we need data to support this assumption. Even if SAH were active *in vivo* and

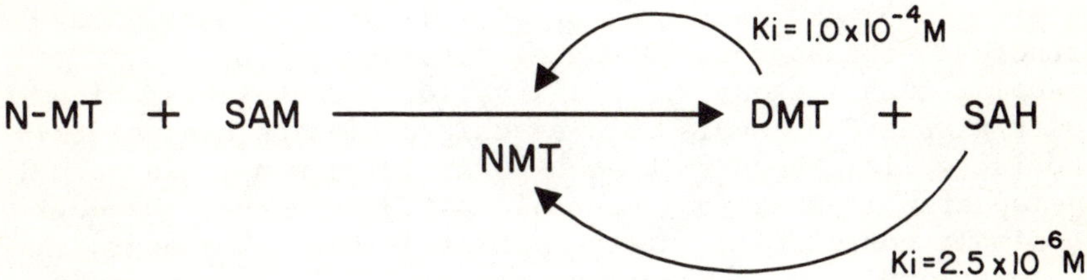

Fig. 4. DMT and especially SAH produce end product inhibition of NTM. Data for the rabbit lung enzyme are given. In our laboratory the Ki for DMT was 1.0 x 10^{-4}M and for SAH 2.5 x 10^{-6}M.

not toxic, one would still be concerned about its stability [for it is enzymatically broken down (Deguchi and Barchas, 1972)] as well as its absorption and penetration through cell membranes and the blood-brain-barrier. Furthermore, SAH is extremely expensive. Hence, it is unlikely that it can be tested in animals for toxicity and specificity of inhibition of methylations *in vivo* in the near future. It is important to find more specific derivatives of SAH and related compounds that are effective NMT inhibitors. Lin *et al*. (1974) have reported that the brains of several animal species, human brain and blood, and bovine pineal gland contain two substances which appear to be small peptides with molecular weights of 600 (I, minor) and 500 (II, major). These findings are especially important to pursue for they indicate other endogenous inhibitors beside SAH which inhibit NMT. Should INMT be selectively inhibited, these substances would indeed be a major breakthrough toward new treatment approaches. Synthetic congeners of such peptides as well as SAH and DMT would be of considerable interest to test as potential selective NMT inhibitors and, if non-toxic, as therapeutic agents. We are actively pursuing this approach.

The use of nicotinic acid and nicotinamide in large doses as treatments for schizophrenia was based upon their ability to be N-methylated and hence to trap excess methyl groups (Hoffer et al., 1957). Baldessarini (1967) has been unable to show that nicotinamide lowers SAM levels in the rat brain. This would be expected for nicotinamide should not readily penetrate the blood-brain-barrier because of its charged form at pH 7.4. The megavitamin approach using this substance unfortunately has not proved effective in the treatment of schizophrenia as reported by the American Psychiatric Association task force on megavitamins (Lipton et al., 1973) and by Lehman et al. (1973) in Canada. Nevertheless, the approach of using alternate substrates for trapping methyl groups is still valid. Some agents which lower tissue SAM levels such as chlorpromazine are antipsychotic, while others such as L-DOPA, imipramine, and pargyline apparently make schizophrenic patients worse. Hence, no simple correlation exists. Nevertheless, this approach is most intriguing. Schatz et al. (1973, 1974) have shown that L-methionine sulfoximine depresses rat brain SAM levels. Perhaps this may explain the curious finding of Heath et al. (1966) that D,L-methionine-d,l-sulfoximine in doses which produce psychotic symptoms and EEG changes in control subjects causes a significant diminution of psychotic symptoms and no EEG changes in chronic schizophrenics. However, just because a compound reduces brain SAM levels does not mean it will be of value in schizophrenics for a reduction in SAM levels can be due to many different mechanisms. For example, SAM synthesis may be reduced or SAM utilization enhanced. Furthermore, toxic methylated metabolites may be formed. Although L-methionine sulfoximine depresses brain SAM, it apparently does not do this by decreased SAM synthesis. Instead, brain histamine methyltransferase and catechol-O-methyl transferase activity are enhanced. Schatz et al. (1974) have suggested that the convulsant actions of methionine sulfoximine may be related to the formation of seizure-inducing methylated products.

Another approach for more effective treatments of schizophrenia would be to enhance the breakdown of hallucinogenic indoles. Most of the hallucinogenic indoles are tertiary amines. Only T is a primary amine. The MAO enzymes are involved in their breakdown, and hence MAO inhibitors should enhance DMT effects. However, Sai-Halász (1963) showed that subjects given 100 mg of iproniazid a day for four days followed by a two-day drug free period had fewer hallucinations and an attenuation of the DMT effect when given DMT on the 7th day. The volunteers did have an odd feeling of a changed personality following DMT which resembled the schizophrenic "wahnstimmung" which precedes the outbreak of a psychosis. In addition, Sai-Halász (1962a,b) showed that 1-methyl-D-lysergic acid butanolamide (Deseril), a 5-HT antagonist, accentuated the experimental psychosis induced by DMT. This investigator felt that by elevating 5-HT brain levels one would protect against DMT hallucinations while blocking 5-HT would enhance the effects of DMT. It is of interest that Wyatt et al. (1972) reported that the administration of 5-HTP to some schizophrenic patients had a beneficial effect. Unfortunately, this was not consistent or reproducible in all schizophrenic patients, indicating a heterogeneity of disease types. There is an obvious discrepancy between the human studies of Sai-Halász and the findings from our own laboratory using animal models of DMT effects. For example, DMT-induced depression of rat shuttle box acquisition is potentiated by iproniazid (Lutz and Domino, 1974). This is shown by a shift to the left in the dose-effect curve of DMT in suppressing one-way acquisition. Similarly, in rats trained for a FR_4 milk reward, single doses of iproniazid potentiate the suppression of DMT-induced bar pressing (Kovacic and Domino, 1973). Pretreatment with iproniazid enhances rat brain and liver levels of DMT (Lu et al., 1974). In addition, DMT induced hyperthermia and pupillary dilatation in the rabbit is also prolonged by iproniazid (Moore et al., 1975). From these animal findings, it would appear that one pathway for the biodegradation of DMT is through MAO. In vitro DMT is a very poor substrate for MAO compared to T (Domino and Krause, 1974b). However, iproniazid in vivo appears to be far better in prolonging rat brain and liver levels of DMT than would be expected from in vitro studies (Lu et al., 1974).

These results, of course, do not rule out a prior demethylation of DMT to T before oxidation by MAO. This possibility is being pursued in our laboratory using demethylase inhibitors. If MAO is important for biotransforming DMT in man, it becomes most intriguing that platelet MAO activity is reduced in schizophrenic patients (Murphy and Wyatt, 1972; Wyatt et al., 1973b; Domino and Sampath-Khanna 1975). Meltzer and Stahl (1974) also measured platelet MAO activity in 12 chronic schizophrenic and 10 acute schizophrenic patients as well as 15 mentally normal controls, using four different substrates. Most of the schizophrenic patients were receiving phenothiazine medication. Meltzer and Stahl felt that this was valid because Murphy and Wyatt found no evidence of any effect of phenothiazines on platelet MAO activity in schizophrenic patients. Both male and female patients were studied. There was a tendency for platelet MAO activity to be greater in female than male controls for the substrates meta-iodobenzylamine, tyramine, and T but not octopamine. Similarly, there was a tendency for platelet MAO activity to be greater in male acute and chronic schizophrenics than in female schizophrenics but the differences were not statistically significant. Since there were no statistical sex differences, the data was combined. Under these circumstances, platelet MAO activity with all four substrates was significantly depressed in the schizophrenic patients compared to the activities in mentally normal controls. In the acute schizophrenic patients, MAO activity was also significantly lower than controls when *meta*-iodobenzylamine and tyramine were employed as substrates. Collins and Sandler (1971) have pointed out that it is not possible to extrapolate the status of human platelet MAO to any other tissue. As discussed above, our own preliminary data would agree in that brain MAO activity is normal using T as the substrate. So far we have obtained from autopsy material the liver of only one chronic schizophrenic patient. In that patient liver MAO activity was normal as well.

The mechanism by which platelet MAO activity is reduced in schizophrenic patients is unclear. It should be noted that there are two basic families of MAO, the A and B types (Yang and Neff, 1974). The A type MAO oxidizes 5-HT and NE, while the B type MAO oxidizes phenethylamine and benzylamine. Amines such as T are oxidized by both types of MAO. Utena *et al*. (1968) determined the regional MAO activity from the brains of five deceased chronic schizophrenic and five cancer patients. They used 5-HT as the substrate, hence they were measuring type A MAO. In the 24 regional brain areas studied they were unable to find any difference between the two groups. However, when the areas were combined into functional brain systems, MAO activity from the schizophrenic patients was lower in all areas except in the cerebral cortex. Vogel *et al*. (1969) used T as the substrate to measure both A and B type MAO activity in the brains of two deceased schizophrenic and three other psychiatric patients. These investigators found no differences in MAO activity in the neocortex of all of the patients, but the schizophrenic patients had low MAO activity in the hypothalamus and caudate. The lowered MAO observed in the caudate of the two schizophrenics is partly consistent with an older study of Birkhäuser (1941) who observed that pallidal MAO activity using tyramine as the substrate was enhanced in two schizophrenic patients over 60 years old. However, in six patients below 60 years at the time of death pallidal MAO activity was decreased below normal ($P < .052$). In our preliminary studies (Domino *et al*., 1973) in which T was used as substrate, there was no difference in MAO activity in 15 regional brain areas of four deceased mentally normal vs. six chronic schizophrenic patients. Similarly, Schwartz et al. (1974a,c) reported that there was no difference in MAO activity using T as substrate in 14 different brain regions of nine schizophrenic and nine mentally normal individuals. Wise and Stein (1973, 1975) also found normal MAO activity in the brains of deceased schizophrenic patients, but dopamine-β-hydroxylase activity was markedly reduced in all brain areas studied. Wyatt et al. (1975b) studied the dopamine-β-hydroxylase activity of postmortem brain specimens from nine chronic schizophrenic patients and nine controls. They were unable to find any statistically significant difference in dopamine-β-hydroxylase activity between the two groups. However, they were able to find a significant negative correlation between the time in the morgue to the time of autopsy and dopamine-β-hydroxylase activity. In addition, there was a significant negative correlation between the dosage of chlorpromazine or its equivalent, and schizophrenic brain dopamine-β-hydroxylase activity. Hence, they suggested that the findings reported by Wise and Stein are secondary to the duration of morgue time to measurement of enzymatic activity and the administration of neuroleptic medication. Dunner et al. (1973) and Wetterberg et al. (1972b) have reported that there is no difference in dopamine-β-hydroxylase activity in the plasma of schizophrenic patients compared to mentally normal controls. In fact, monozygotic twins discordant for schizophrenia, whose dopamine-β-hydroxylase activity was in the normal range, showed a high correlation between twin pairs, indicating that plasma dopamine-β-hydroxylase activity is under genetic control, an observation suggested by many others for various diseases (Weinshilboum and Axelrod, 1971; Lieberman et al., 1972; Wetterberg et al., 1972a; Wooton et al., 1973).

In addition to the numerous variables associated with studying brain tissue of cadavers, MAO activity has been reported to be positively correlated with age (Birkhäuser, 1941; Robinson et al., 1972). It is reasonable to conclude that there seems to be no significant alteration in schizophrenic brain MAO activity, although more detailed studies using selective type A or B substrates and inhibitors are indicated. Recently, Schwartz et al. (1974b) extended their initial studies and characterized human platelet MAO activity as primarily type B. In their studies of autopsy material, they showed that both type A and type B MAO were found distributed throughout the brain. There were no significant differences in MAO A and MAO B activity between the brains of eight chronic schizophrenics and nine mentally normal individuals.

These predominantly negative results for brain MAO are in marked contrast to the findings that chronic schizophrenic patients as a group have a marked reduction in type B MAO activity in platelets compared to mentally normal controls, as described above. It should be noted that normal monozygotic and dizygotic twins have a high inheritability for platelet MAO activity (Nies *et al*., 1973). Similarly, platelet type B MAO activity in 13 monozygotic twin pairs discordant for schizophrenia shows a high correlation between twins (Wyatt *et al*., 1973b). Low platelet MAO activity in the schizophrenic twins was mirrored by similarly low activity in their phenotypically normal co-twins. These investigators interpreted their findings that low platelet type B MAO activity is associated with a diathesis toward schizophrenia and not secondary in some way to this condition. It seems most crucial to study the MAO activity of other tissues of schizophrenic patients to determine the generality of this deficit in peripheral type B MAO activity. It is not known whether type A or type B MAO oxidizes DMT. This has obvious implications for treatments which can facilitate MAO activity and may be beneficial for schizophrenic patients.

Garrelis *et al*. (1975) determined the blood concentrations of 5-HT in chronic unmedicated schizophrenic patients. In comparison to mentally normal controls, whole blood 5-HT was significantly higher in the patients as a group. Mean whole blood 5-HT was 186 ng/ml for the control subjects and 232 ng/ml for the schizophrenic patients ($P < .05$). This difference remained significant when corrections for platelet counts were made. However, when the patients were divided into medicated and unmedicated groups, the elevation in 5-HT occurred primarily in the drug-free group. Mean whole blood 5-HT was 298 ng/ml for the drug-free patients compared with 199 ng/ml for the patients receiving psychotropic medication ($P < .01$). Patients on drugs did not differ significantly from the controls. These differences could not be explained on the basis of age or platelet counts. The findings of high blood 5-HT concentrations in drug-free schizophrenic patients is consistent with the observations described above that MAO activity is low in the platelets of such patients (Murphy and Wyatt, 1972; Wyatt *et al*., 1973b). It is not certain whether these two parameters are related in a cause and effect manner. There are obviously many factors which influence blood and platelet 5-HT concentrations. Inasmuch as most of the 5-HT in blood is in the platelets, it suggests that the platelets are the primary problem. Obviously, the 5-HT concentrations of platelets can be influenced by the rate of synthesis of 5-HT, its entry into the blood stream, plasma and platelet MAO activity and the functional status of uptake, storage and release mechanisms in platelets. It is well known that 5-HT is only one of many amines biotransformed by platelet MAO. Furthermore, platelet MAO is primarily of the B type, as described previously and hence 5-HT is not a very good substrate for this enzyme. Other studies reported in the literature describing blood 5-HT levels in chronic schizophrenics have been controversial (Jus et al., 1958; Feldstein et al., 1959; Todrick et al., 1960; Halevy et al., 1965) because of the problem of possible drug effects, age matching and platelet count differences. The findings of elevated blood 5-HT concentrations in chronic unmedicated schizophrenics as reported by Garrellis et al. have an analogy to the findings of high 5-HT blood levels in children suffering from early infantile autism (Ritvo et al., 1970).

Another approach to a new treatment is to enhance DMT biotransformation. There are several other theoretical pathways by which DMT and related indole hallucinogens can be biotransformed. These include demethylation, N-oxide formation and hydroxylation. In view of the essential role of the liver microsomal enzymes in these metabolic reactions, it would be of considerable interest to study the effects of inhibitors of drug metabolism such as SKF-525A or liver microsomal enzyme inducers such as phenobarbital on the behavioral effects of DMT as well as on tissue levels of this substance. By selectively enhancing the breakdown of DMT and related indoles, one might be able to develop a novel treatment.

Still another approach is to find more effective DMT antagonists. Although chlorpromazine antagonizes the hyperthermia, pupillary dilatation and behavioral excitation of DMT in the rabbit, other neuroleptic agents having anti-5-HT actions such as methiothepin (Monachon et al., 1972) are more effective (Moore et al., 1974). DeFrance et al. (1975) also found methiothepin to antagonize the effects of DMT and related indole alkylamines (but not 5-HT) on the cat hippocampal-septal circuit. Recently, we have found that methiothepin also blocks the depressant effects of DMT at the lateral geniculate nucleus of the cat (Moore et al., 1974). More selective agents should be developed for methiothepin blocks DA, NE, and 5-HT receptors (Lloyd and Bartholini, 1974). It is important to develop selective antagonists of indole hallucinogens and such studies are currently proceeding in our laboratory at the Lafayette Clinic.

Conclusion. There are many new therapeutic approaches

possible based upon the indole hallucinogen hypothesis. They seem worthy to pursue.

V. What is the role of animal models in seeking new treatments of schizophrenia based upon the indole hallucinogen hypothesis? If indole hallucinogens exist in some schizophrenic patients and are psychotogenic, then the use of animal models to find new treatments is of considerable value. Some of the possible approaches already have been discussed. Nevertheless, it may be of value to review them further as per the topic of this symposium.

Obviously, one of the major problems of finding an antagonist of a hallucinogen is to quantify hallucinations in animals. Yet this is impossible. No one can ever determine if an animal hallucinates. We can only study behavioral, chemical and physiological endpoints. Let us consider some of the behavioral measures. They fall into two broad categories. 1) Those that are behaviorally disrupting and nonspecific, and 2) those behaviors that are specifically related to hallucinogens. Various behavioral endpoints can be used to determine the disruptive effects of indole hallucinogens. One which we have used is one-way shuttle box acquisition to an electric shock (Tenen, 1966; Caldwell *et al.*, 1970). DMT produces a dose-related suppression of avoidance acquisition in this task. The advantage of this behavior is that it is rapidly acquired; hence, naive animals can be run the same day. Its disadvantage is that it is rather insensitive to DMT and nonspecific. Another nonspecific task which lends itself to the study of the duration of action of hallucinogens is suppression of fixed ratio responding for a food reward. We have used a FR_4 schedule for sweetened milk reinforcement in rats food-deprived to maintain 70% of optimal weight. Such animals can easily be trained to bar press for food. The administration of DMT and related substances produces an abrupt cessation of operant responding and abrupt recovery. Hence, the duration of action of the hallucinogen can be measured as the period of non-responding. A large variety of other operant behaviors could also be used. However, drugs which are potential antagonists must in themselves not affect such behaviors. Otherwise, they cannot be tested as suitable antagonists. In addition, many operant behaviors are nonspecific. Psychomotor stimulants, for example, may also suppress responding. One of the problems highlighted by the administration of a potential antagonist is that with the two behaviors used in our laboratory, chlorpromazine has only been able to potentiate the actions of *d*-amphetamine and not antagonize them as is generally known for other behaviors. This may simply be a dose-related phenomenon for small doses of chlorpromazine prolong amphetamine-induced stereotypes as well as other behavioral effects (Borella et al., 1969; Lal and Sourkes, 1972). Inasmuch as larger doses of chlorpromazine reduce behavioral responding, nonspecific behaviors are very limited in testing for antagonists of hallucinogenic activity. Appel (1968) has reviewed extensively the effects of psychotomimetic drugs, especially LSD-25, on animal behavior. Other behavioral models he has referred to can probably be very useful to screen potential antagonists.

A biochemical measure which can be used to test for indole hallucinogens of the LSD-25 type is an apparent reduction in brain 5-HT turnover. Brain 5-HT increases and 5-HIAA decreases following LSD and related compounds (Aghajanian and Freedman, 1968). Inasmuch as MAO inhibitors do the same, one must be certain MAO inhibition is not involved. Hence, the endpoint is nonspecific. Another nonspecific biochemical endpoint for indole hallucinogen effect is brain cyclic AMP. Uzunov and Weiss (1972) have shown that 3 μmol/kg of LSD and especially 0.1 mmol/kg of DMT given i.p. elevates rat cerebral cyclic AMP levels. Trifluoperazine both in vitro and in vivo antagonized the increase induced by these two hallucinogens. Inasmuch as these substituted phenothiazines are not very effective in antagonizing all of the behavioral and electrophysiologic effects of DMT, one wonders about the specificity of this antagonism.

Physiologic endpoints such as temperature elevation and pupillary dilatation can also be used for assaying hallucinogenic activity. It is well known that hallucinogens of the LSD-25 type elevate the rectal temperature of rabbits (Rothlin, 1957). Although hyperthermia is a nonspecific endpoint, it can be used for determining potential antagonistic effects. In this animal test, both chlorpromazine and methiothepin are effective antagonists of DMT-induced hypothermia and pupillary dilatation, as mentioned above (Moore et al., 1975). Again, this test suffers from lack of specificity inasmuch as psychomotor stimulants also elevate rectal temperature. Furthermore, with α-methyl-para-tyrosine one can dissociate LSD-induced increase in rectal temperature from its other behavioral effects which are reduced (Horita and Hamilton, 1969).

More specific tests of hallucinogenic activity include head bobbing in mice (Corne and Pickering, 1967; Siegel and Jarvik, 1972), splayed legs in rodents (personal observations), or splayed wings in chicks (Mandell et al., 1971). To my knowledge, these endpoints have not been widely used for studying hallucingen antagonists. However, T convulsions have been used as an endpoint in rats for studying potential 5-HT antagonists (Tedeschi et al., 1959). Bovet-Gatti profiles based upon the distribution of premature, optimal or late responses on rat bar-pressing behavior to avoid electroshock have also been suggested as an excellent way of screening for hallucinogens including DMT (Gatti and Bovet, 1963; Gatti, 1964; Bovet and Gatti, 1965; Smythies, 1970). Smythies et al. (1972) have reported that N,N-diethyl butyramide (DBA) blocks the effects of DMT using this technique.

One can also use various neurophysiologic endpoints for screening potential antagonists of hallucinogens such as LSD-25 (Koella, 1968). Inasmuch as LSD-25 and indole hallucinogens block the lateral geniculate evoked response (Evarts et al., 1955; Bishop et al., 1958, 1959; Evarts 1958), one can use this response as a test of potential antagonists, using the cat or monkey with acute or chronic indwelling brain electrodes. This approach suffers in that it is not a suitable rapid screening procedure. Either acute animals must be used under general anesthesia or chronic animals who move about and are likely to show more variability. Another approach with similar limitations is to measure the rate of firing of the serotonergic neurons in the raphé nucleus. After LSD-25 and mescaline, the firing rates are reduced (Aghajanian et al., 1970b). Similarly, DMT has been shown to reduce raphé neuron firing (Aghajanian et al., 1970a).

Conclusion: As yet there are no satisfactory animal models for studying indole hallucinogen antagonists. Most are either nonspecific or very time consuming. Should DMT and related agents be shown to be psychotogenic even in a minority of schizophrenics, it will behoove us all to use such animal models to a maximum.

Acknowledgements

The author would like to acknowledge a most remarkable psychiatrist and friend, Dr. Jacques Gottlieb, who made this research possible. Hopefully, the ideas expressed will provide eventually some better treatments of schizophrenia. In addition, the personnel of the Pharmacology Laboratory, whose research is described, have provided some of the data upon which this manuscript is based.

References

Adams, R.L.P.: Delayed methylation of DNA in developing sea urchin embryos. Nature (New Biol.) 244: 27-29, 1973.

Aghajanian, G.K. and Freedman, D.X.: Biochemical and morphological aspects of LSD pharmacology. In Psychopharmacology - A Review of Progress 1957-1967, ed. by D.H. Efron, pp. 1185-1193 PHSP #1836, Superintendent of Documents, Washington, D.C., 1968.

Aghajanian, G.K., Foote, W.F. and Sheard, M.H.: Action of psychotogenic drugs on single midbrain raphé neurons. J. Pharmacol. Exp. Ther. 171: 178-187, 1970a.

Aghajanian, G.K., Sheard, M.H. and Foote, W.E.: LSD and mescaline: Comparison of effects on single units in the midbrain raphé. In Psychotomimetic Drugs, ed. by D.H. Efron, pp. 165-170, Raven Press, New York, 1970b.

Ahn, H.S., Walker, R.W., VandenHeuvel, W.J.A., Rosegay, A. and Mandel, L.R.: Studies on the in vivo biosynthesis of N,N-dimethyltryptamine (DMT) in the rabbit and rat. Fed. Proc. 32: 511, 1973.

Alexander, F., Curtis, G.C., III, Sprince, H. and Crosley, A.P., Jr.: L-Methionine and L-tryptophan feedings in non-psychotic and schizophrenic patients with and without tranylcypromine. J. Nerv. Ment. Dis. 137: 135-142, 1963.

Appel, J.B.: The effects of "psychotomimetic" drugs on animal behavior. In Pharmacology - A Review of Progress 1957-1967, ed. by D.H. Efron, pp. 1211-1222, PHSP #1836, Superintendent of Documents, Washington, D.C., 1968.

Axelrod, J.: The enzymatic N-methylation of serotonin and other amines. J. Pharmacol. Exp. Ther. 138: 28-33, 1962.

Baldessarini, R.J.: Factors influencing S-adenosylmethionine levels in mammalian tissue. In Amines and Schizophrenia, ed. by H.E. Himwich, S.S. Kety and J.R. Smythies, pp. 199-207, Pergamon Press, New York, 1967.

Baldessarini, R.J. and Kopin, I.J.: S-Adenosylmethionine in brain and other tissues. J. Neurochem. 13: 769-777, 1966.

Ban, R.: Monoamine oxidase inhibitor antidepressants, Chapt. 15. In Psychopharmacology, by T. Ban, pp. 290-312, The Williams and Wilkins Co., Baltimore, 1969.

Banerjee, S.P. and Snyder, S.H.: Methyltetrahydrofolic acid mediates N- and O-methylation of biogenic amines. Science 182: 74-75, 1973.

Barchas, J.D., Elliott, G.R., DoAmaral, J., Erdelyi, E., O'Connor, S., Bowden, M., Brodie, H.K.H., Berger, P.A., Renson, J. and Wyatt, R.J.: Triptolines: Formation from tryptamines and 5-MTHF by human platelets. Arch. Gen. Psychiat. 31: 862-867, 1974.

Benington, F., Morin, R.D. and Clark, L.C.: 5-Methoxy, N,N-dimethyltryptamine, a possible endogenous psychotoxin. Alabama J. Med. Sci. 2: 397-403, 1965.

Bidder, T.G., Mandel, L.R., Ahn, H.S., Walker, R.W. and VandenHeuvel, W.J.A.: Blood and urinary dimethyltryptamine in acute psychotic disorders. Lancet 1: 165, 1974.

Birkhäuser, H.: Cholinesterase und mono-aminoxydase im centralen nervensystem. Schweiz. med. Wochenschr. 71: 750-752, 1941.

Bishop, P.O., Burke, W. and Hayhow, W.R.: Lysergic acid diethylamide block of lateral geniculate synapses and relief by repetitive stimulation. Exp. Neurol. 1: 556-568, 1959.

Bishop, P.O., Field, G., Hennessy, B.L. and Smith, J.R.: Actions of D-lysergic acid diethylamide on lateral geniculate synapses. J. Neurophysiol. 21: 529-549, 1958.

Borella, L., Herr, F. and Wojdan, A.: Prolongation of certain effects of amphetamine by chlorpromazine. Canad. J. Physiol. and Pharmacol. 47: 7-13, 1969.

Bovet, D. and Gatti, G.L.: Pharmacology of instrumental avoidance conditioning. In Proceedings of 2nd International Pharmacological Meeting, pp. 75-89, Prague, 1965.

Caldwell, D.F., Oberleas, D., Clancy, J.J. and Prasad, A.S.: Behavioral impairment in adult rats following acute zinc deficiency. Proc. Soc. Exp. Biol. Med. 133: 1417-1421, 1970.

Cohen, I. and Vogel, W.H.: Determination and physiological disposition of dimethyltryptamine and diethyltryptamine in rat brain, liver and plasma. Biochem. Pharmacol. 21: 1214-1216, 1972.

Cole, J.O., Freedman, A.M. and Friedhoff, A.J.: Psychopathology and Psychopharmacology. Johns Hopkins Univ. Press, Baltimore, 1973.

Collins, G.G.S. and Sandler, M.: Human platelet monoamine oxidase. Biochem. Pharmacol. 20: 289-296, 1971.

Connell, P.H.: Amphetamine Psychosis, p. 133. Chapman and Hall, Ltd., London, 1958.

Corne, S.J. and Pickering, R.W.: A possible correlation between drug-induced hallucinations in man and a behavioral response in mice. Psychopharmacologia 11: 65-78, 1967.

Coward, J.K., D'Urso-Scott, M. and Sweet, W.D.: Inhibition of catechol-O-methyltransferase by S-adenosylhomocysteine and S-adenosylhomocysteine sulfoxide, a potential transition-state analog. Biochem. Pharmacol. 21: 1200-1203, 1972.

Dagley, S. and Nicholson, D.E.: An Introduction to Metabolic Pathways. John Wiley & Sons, New York, 1970.

DeFrance, J.F., McCrea, R.A. and Yosihara, H.: Effects of certain indole amines in the hippocampal-septal circuit. Exper. Neurol. In press, 1975.

Deguchi, T. and Barchas, J.: Inhibition of transmethylations of biogenic amines by S-adenosylhomocysteine. J. Biol. Chem. 246: 3175-3181, 1972.

Domino, E.F.: Pharmacological analysis of the pathobiology of schizophrenia. In Schizophrenia, Current Concepts in Research, ed. by D.V.S. Sankar, pp. 148-160, PJD Publications Ltd., Hickville, N.Y., 1969.

Domino, E.F., Krause, R.R. and Bowers, J.: Various enzymes involved with putative neurotransmitters--regional distribution in the brain of deceased mentally normal, chronic schizophrenics or organic brain sydrome patients. Arch. Gen. Psychiat. 29: 195-201, 1973.

Domino, E.F. and Krause, R.R.: Plasma tryptophan tolerance curves in drug free normal controls, schizophrenic patients and prisoner volunteers. J. Psychiat. Res. 10: 247-261, 1974a.

Domino, E.F. and Krause, R.R.: Unpublished observations, 1974b.

Domino, E.F. and Luby, E.D.: Abnormal mental states induced by phencyclidine as a model of schizophrenia. Chapt. 3. In Psychopathology and Psychopharmacology, ed. by J.O. Cole, A. Friedhoff and A.M. Friedman, pp. 35-50, Proc. 62nd Meeting of Amer. Psychopath. Assoc., Johns Hopkins Press, Baltimore, 1973.

Domino, E.F. and Sampath-Khanna, S.: Reduced blood platelet monoamine oxidase activity in unmedicated chronic schizophrenic patients. Am. J. Psychiat. Accepted for publication, 1975.

Dunner, D.L., Cohn, C.K., Weinshilboum, R.M. and Wyatt, R.J.: The activity of dopamine-beta-hydroxylase and methionine-activating enzyme in blood of schizophrenic patients. Biol. Psychiat. 6: 215-220, 1973.

Ellinwood, E.H., Jr.: Amphetamine psychosis: A multi-dimensional process. Seminars in Psychiat. 1: 208-226, 1969.

Ellinwood, E.H., Jr. and Sudilovsky, A.: Chronic amphetamine intoxication: Behavioral model of psychoses. Chapt. 4. In Psychopathology and Psychopharmacology, ed. by J.O. Cole, A. Friedhoff and A.M. Friedman, pp. 51-78, Proc. 62nd Meeting of Amer. Psychopath. Assoc., Johns Hopkins Press, Baltimore, 1973.

Evarts, E.V.: Effects of a series of indoles on synaptic transmission in the lateral geniculate nucleus of the cat. In Progress in Neurobiology III -- Psychopharmacology, ed. by H.H. Pennes, pp. 173-194, Hoeber-Harper, New York, 1958.

Evarts, E.V., Landau, W., Freygang, W., Jr. and Marshall, W.H.: Some effects of lysergic acid diethylamide and bufotenine on electrical activity in the cat's visual system. Am. J. Physiol. 182: 594-598, 1955.

Fabing, H.D.: On going berserk: A neurochemical inquiry. Amer. J. Psychiat. 113: 409-415, 1956.

Fabing, H.D. and Hawkins, R.: Intravenous bufotenin injection in human beings. Science 123: 886-887, 1956.

Feldstein, A., Hoagland, H. and Freeman, H.: Blood and urinary serotonin and 5-hydroxyindole acetic acid levels in schizophrenic patients and normal subjects. J. Nerv. Ment. Dis. 129: 62-68, 1959.

Fernstrom, J.D. and Wurtman, R.J.: Nutrition and the brain. Scientific American 230: 84-91, 1974.

Fisher, R.: Chemistry of the brain. Nature (Lond.) 220: 411-412, 1968.

Franzen, Fr. and Gross, H.: Tryptamine, N,N-dimethyltryptamine, N,N-dimethyl-5-hydroxytryptamine and 5-methoxytryptamine in human blood and urine. Nature (Lond.) 206: 1052, 1965.

Frohman, C.E.: Plasma proteins and schizophrenia. In Biological Psychiatry, ed. by J. Mendels, pp. 131-148, John Wiley & Sons, Inc., New York, 1973.

Gaitonde, M.K.: Sulfur amino acids. Chapt. 8 in Handbook of Neurochemistry, Vol. III, ed. by A. Lajtha, pp. 225-287. Plenum Press, New York, 1970.

Garattini, S. and Valzelli, L.: Serotonin. Elsevier Publishing Co., Amsterdam, 1965.

Garrelis, E., Gillin, J.C., Wyatt, R.J. and Neff, N.: Elevated blood serotonin concentrations in chronic, unmedicated schizophrenics: A preliminary study. Am. J. Psychiat. 132: 184-186, 1975.

Gatti, G.L.: Analysis of parameters of the action of psycholeptic and psychomimetic drugs in a lever-pressing avoidance conditioning. In Neuropsychopharmacology, ed. by P.B. Bradley, F. Flügel and P. Hoch, pp. 514-518, Elsevier, Amsterdam, 1964.

Gatti, G.L. and Bovet, D.: Analysis of the action of the psychotropic drugs in a "lever-pressing avoidance" conditioning. In Psychopharmacological Methods, ed. by Z. Votava, M. Horvath, and O. Vinar, pp. 50-51, Pergamon Press, Oxford, 1973.

Gessner, P.K. and Page, I.H.: Behavioral effects of 5-methoxy N,N-dimethyltryptamine, other tryptamines and LSD. Am. J. Physiol. 203: 167-172, 1962.

Gillin, J.C., Cannon, E., Magyar, R., Schwartz, M. and Wyatt, R.J.: Failure of N,N-dimethyltryptamine to evoke tolerance in cats. Biol. Psychiat. 7: 213-220, 1973.

Gilmour, D.G., Manowitz, P., Frosch, W.A. and Shopsin, B.: Association of plasma tryptophan levels with clinical change in female schizophrenic patients. Biol. Psychiat. 6: 119-128, 1973.

Gottlieb, J.S. and Frohman, C.E.: Towards a biological mechanism in schizophrenia. In Biological Mechanisms of Schizophrenia and Schizophrenia-like Psychoses, ed. by H. Mitsuda and T. Fukuda, pp. 156-166, Igaku-shoin Ltd., Tokyo, 1974.

Greenberg, R.: N,N-dimethylated and N,N-diethylated indoleamines in schizophrenia. In Chemical Modulation of Brain Function -- A Tribute to J.E.P. Toman, ed. by H.C. Sabelli, pp. 277-296, Raven Press, New York, 1973.

Gross, V.H. and Franzen, Fr.: Zur bestimmung korpereigener amine in biologischen substraten. Zeitschrift für Klinische Chemie 3: 99-102, 1965.

Guroff, G. and Lovenberg, W.: Metabolism of aromatic amino acids. Chapt. 7. In Handbook of Neurochemistry, Vol. III, ed. by A. Lajtha, pp. 209-223, Plenum Press, New York, 1970.

Halevy, A., Moos, R.H. and Solomon, G.F.: A relationship between blood serotonin concentrations and behavior in psychiatric patients. J. Psychiat. Res. 3: 1-10, 1965.

Heath, R.G., Nesselhof, W., Jr., Bishop, M.P. and Byers, L.W.: Behavioral and metabolic changes associated with administration of tetraethylthiuram disulfide. Dis. Nerv. System 26: 99-106, 1965.

Heath, R.G., Nesselhof, W., Jr. and Timmons, E.: D,L-Methionine-d,l-sulfoximine effects in schizophrenic patients. Arch. Gen. Psychiat. 14: 213-217, 1966.

Heller, B.: N-Methylating enzyme in blood of schizophrenics. Psychosomatics 12: 273-274, 1971.

Himwich, H.E. (ed.): Biochemistry, Schizophrenias and Affective Illnesses. Williams and Wilkins Co., Baltimore, 1971.

Himwich, H.E., Kety, S.S., and Smythies, J.R. (eds.): Amines and Schizophrenia. Pergamon Press, Oxford, 1967.

Himwich, H.E., Narasimhachari, S., Heller, B., Spaide, J., Haskovec, L., Fujimori, M. and Tabushi, K.: Biochemical approaches to the study of schizophrenia. In Chemical Modulation of Brain Function -- A Tribute to J.E.P. Toman, ed. by H.C. Sabelli, pp. 297-311, Raven Press, New York, 1973.

Hoffer, A., Osmond, H., Callbeck, M.J. and Kahan, I.: Treatment of schizophrenia with nicotinic acid and nicotinamide. J. Clin. Exp. Psychopath. 18: 131-158, 1957.

Holmstedt, B. and Lindgren, J.B.: Chemical constituents and pharmacology of South American snuffs. In Ethnopharmacologic Search for Psychoactive Drugs, ed. by D.H. Efron, pp. 339-382, Publication #1645, Public Health Service, Washington, D.C., 1967.

Horita, A. and Hamilton, A.E.: Lysergic acid diethylamide: Dissociation of its behavioral and hyperthermic actions by DL-alpha-methyl-p-tyrosine. Science 164: 78-79, 1969.

Hsu, L.L. and Mandell, A.J.: Multiple N-methyltransferases for aromatic alkylamines in brain. Life Sci. 13: 847-858, 1973.

Isbell, H.: Quoted in Ethnopharmacologic Search for Psychoactive Drugs, ed. by D.H. Efron, p. 369, Publication #1645, Public Health Service, Washington, D.C., 1967.

Jaccarini, A. and Jepson, J.B.: The 6-hydroxylation of tryptamines by microsomal preparations from human liver tissue obtained at routine autopsy. Experientia 24: 29, 1968.

Jus, A., Laskowska, D. et Zimny, S.: Recherches sur le comportement de la serotonine dans le serum snaguin des schizophrenes. Annales Medico-Psychologiques. 116: 898-913, 1958.

Kaplan, J., Mandel, L.R., Walker, R.W., VandenHeuvel, W. J.A., Stillman, R., Gillin, J.C. and Wyatt, R.J.: Blood and urine levels of N,N-dimethyltryptamine following administration of psychoactive dosages to human subjects. Psychopharmacologia 38: 239-245, 1974a.

Kaplan, J., Stillman, R.C., Gillin, J.C. and Wyatt, R.J.: Attempts to evoke tolerance to DMT in man. New Research Abstracts, p. 3, American Psychiatric Association Meeting, Detroit, May, 1974b.

Kerr, S.J.: Competing methyltransferase systems. J. Biol. Chem. 247: 4248-4252, 1972.

Kety, S.S.: Current biochemical approaches to schizophrenia. New England J. Med. 276: 325-331, 1967.

Koella, W.P.: Invited discussion of Dr. J. Appel's paper: Neurophysiological effects of psychotomimetic substances (A supplemental review). In Psychopharmacology--A Review of Progress 1957-1967, ed. by D.H. Efron, pp. 1223-1230, PHSP #1836, Superintendent of Documents, Washington, D.C., 1968.

Koella, W.P., Beaulieu, R.F. and Bergen, J.R.; Stereotyped behavior and cyclic changes in response produced by LSD in goats. Int. J. Neuropharmacol. 3: 397-403, 1964.

Korevaar, W.C., Geyer, M.A., Knapp, S., Hsu, L.L. and Mandell, A.J.: Regional distribution of 5-methyltetrahydrofolic acid in brain. Nature (New Biol.) 245: 244-245, 1973.

Kovacic, B. and Domino, E.F.: Effects of various drugs on DMT-induced disruption of rat bar pressing behavior. The Pharmacologist 15: 218, 1973.

Kovacic, B. and Domino, E.F.: Tolerance to behavioral effects of dimethyltryptamine (DMT) in the rat. Fed. Proc. 33: 549, 1974.

Krause, R.R. and Domino, E.F.: Kinetics of product inhibition of rabbit lung N-methyltransferase. Res. Comm. Chem. Pathol. and Pharmacol. 9(2): 359-374, 1974.

Lal, S. and Sourkes, R.L.: Effect of various chlorpromazine metabolites in amphetamine-induced stereotyped behavior in the rat. Europ. J. Pharmacol. 17: 283-286, 1972.

Lehmann, H.E., Ban, T.A. and Ananth, J.V.: Nicotinic acid and the transmethylation hypothesis of schizophrenia. Chapt. 14. In Psychopathology and Psychopharmacology, ed. by J.O. Cole, A. Friedhoff, pp. 219-230, Proc. 62nd Meeting of Amer. Psychopath. Assoc., Johns Hopkins Press, Baltimore, 1973.

Lewis, G.P. (ed.): Symposium on 5-Hydroxytryptamine. Pergamon Press, London, 1958.

Lieberman, A.N., Freedman, L.S. and Goldstein, M.: Serum dopamine-β-hydroxylase activity in patients with Huntington's chorea and Parkinson's disease. Lancet 1: 153-154, 1972.

Lin, R.L. and Narasimhachari, N.: Evidence for the absence of amine-N-methylation and O-methylation in indoleethylamines with methyltetrahydrofolic acid dependent N-methyltransferase. Res. Comm. Chem. Path. and Pharmacol. 8: 535-542, 1974.

Lin, R.L., Narasimhachari, N. and Himwich, H.E.: Inhibition of indolethylamine-N-methyltransferase by S-adenosylhomocysteine. Biochem. Biophys. Res. Comm. 54: 751-759, 1973.

Lin, R.L., Narasimhachari, N. and Himwich, H.E.: Specific endogenous inhibitors for indolethylamine-N-methyltransferase. Trans. Am. Soc. Neurochem. 5: 156, 1974.

Lipinski, J., Mandel, L.R., Ahn, H.S., VandenHeuvel, W.J. A. and Walker, R.W.: Blood dimethyltryptamine concentrations in psychotic disorders. Biol. Psychiat. 9: 89-91, 1974.

Lipton, M.A., Ban, T.A., Kane, L.J., Levine, J., Mosher, L.R. and Wittenborn, R.: Megavitamin and orthomolecular therapy in psychiatry. A report of the APA Task Force on vitamin therapy in psychiatry. Task Force Report 7. American Psychiatric Association, Washington, D.C., July, 1973.

Lloyd, K.G. and Bartholini, G.: The effect of methiothepin on cerebral monoamine neurons. Advances in Biochemical Psychopharmacology 10: 305-309, Serotonin - New Vistas, ed. by E. Costa, G.L. Gessa and M. Sandler. Raven Press, New York, 1974.

Lu, L.J., Wilson, A.E., Moore, R.H. and Domino, E.F.: Correlation between brain N,N-dimethyltryptamine (DMT) levels and bar pressing behavior in rats: Effect of MAO inhibition. The Pharmacologist 16: 237, 1974.

Lutz, M.P. and Domino, E.F.: Unpublished observations, 1974.

Mandel, L.R.: Personal Communication, 1974.

Mandel, L.R.: Dimethyltryptamine: Its biosynthesis and possible role in mental disease. In Neurotransmitter Balances Regulating Behavior, ed. by E.F. Domino and J. Davis, Ann Arbor, Michigan, 1975.

Mandel, L.R., Ahn, H.S., VandenHeuvel, W.J.A. and Walker, R.W.: Indoleamine-N-methyltransferase in human lung. Biochem. Pharmacol. 21: 1197-1200, 1972.

Mandel, L.R., Rosenzweig, S. and Kuehl, F.A., Jr.: Purification and substrate specificity of indoleamine-N-methyltransferase. Biochem. Pharmacol. 21: 712-716, 1971.

Mandel, L.R., Rosegay, A., Walker, R.W., VandenHeuvel, W.J.A. and Rokach, J.: 5-Methyltetrahydrofolate acid as a mediator in the formation of pyridoindoles. Science 186: 741-743, 1974.

Mandell, A.J., Buckingham, B. and Segal, D.: Behavioral, metabolic, and enzymatic studies of a brain indole-ethylamine N-methylating system. In Brain Chemistry and Mental Disease, ed. by B.T. Ho and W. McIsaac, pp. 37-60, Plenum Press, New York, 1971.

Mandell, A.J. and Morgan, M.: Indole(ethyl)amine N-methyltransferase in human brain. Nature (New Biol.) 230: 85-87, 1971.

Manowitz, P., Gilmour, D.G. and Racevskis, J.: Low plasma tryptophan levels in recently hospitalized schizophrenics. Biol. Psychiat. 6: 109-118, 1973.

Martin, W.R. and Sloan, J.W.: Effects of infused tryptamine in man. Psychopharmacologia 18: 231-237, 1970.

Martin, W.R., Sloan, J.W., Christian, S.T. and Clements, T.H.: Brain levels of tryptamine. Psychopharmacologia 24: 331-346, 1972.

McIsaac, W.M.: A biochemical concept of mental disease. Post Grad. Med. 30: 111-118, 1961a.

McIsaac, W.M.: Formation of 1-methyl-6-methoxy-1,2,3,4-tetrahydro-2-carboline under physiological conditions. Biochim. Biophys. Acta 52: 607-609, 1961b.

Meltzer, H.Y. and Stahl, S.M.: Platelet monoamine oxidase activity and substrate preferences in schizophrenic patients. Research Communications Chem. Path. and Pharmacol. 7: 419-431, 1974.

Monachon, M.A., Burkard, W.P., Jalfre, M. and Haefely, W.: Blockade of central 5-hydroxytryptamine receptors by methiothepin. Naunyn-Schmiedeberg's Arch. Pharmakol. 274: 192-197, 1972.

Morgan, M. and Mandell, A.J.: Indole(ethyl)amine N-methyltransferase in the brain. Science 165: 492-493, 1969.

Moore, R.H., Demetriou, S.K. and Domino, E.F.: Effects of iproniazid, chlorpromazine and methiothepin on DMT induced changes in body temperature, pupil dilatation, blood pressure and EEG in the rabbit. Arch. Int. Pharmacodyn. et Ther. 213: 64-72, 1975.

Moore, R.H., Hatada, K. and Domino, E.F.: Effects of N,N-dimethyltryptamine (DMT) alone and after pretreatment with methiothepin, chlorpromazine or haloperidol on evoked potentials in the visual system of the cat. Soc. for Neurosciences, 4th Annual Meeting, St. Louis, p. 471, 1974.

Murphree, H.B., Dippy, R.H., Jenney, E.H. and Pfeiffer, C.C.: Effects in normal man of α-methyltryptamine and α-ethyltryptamine. Clin. Pharmacol. Ther. 2: 722-726, 1961.

Murphy, D.L. and Wyatt, R.J.: Reduced monoamine oxidase activity in blood platelets from schizophrenic patients. Nature (Lond.) 238: 225-226, 1972.

Narasimhachari, N., Baumann, P., Pak, H.S., Carpenter, W. T., Zocchi, A.F., Hokanson, L., Fujimori, M. and Himwich, H.E.: Gas chromatographic-mass spectrometric identification of urinary bufotenin and dimethyltryptamine in drug-free chronic schizophrenic patients. Biol. Psychiat. 8: 293-305, 1974.

Narasimhachari, N., Heller, B., Spaide, J., Haskovec, L., Fujimori, M., Tabushi, K. and Himwich, H.E.: Urinary studies of schizophrenics and controls. Biol. Psychiat. 3: 9-20, 1971a.

Narasimhachari, N., Heller, B., Spaide, J., Haskovec, L., Meltzer, H., Strahilevitz, M. and Himwich, H.E.: N,N-dimethylated indoleamines in blood. Biol. Psychiat. 3: 21-23, 1971b.

Narasimhachari, N., Plaut, J.M. and Himwich, H.E.: Indoleethylamine-N-methyltransferase in serum samples of schizophrenics and normal controls. Life Sci. 11, Part 2: 221-227, 1972.

Nies, A., Robinson, D.S., Lamborn, K.R. and Lampert, R.P.: Genetic control of platelet and plasma monoamine oxidase activity. Arch. Gen. Psychiat. 28: 834-838, 1973.

Randrup, A., Munkvad, I. and Usden, P.: Adrenergic mechanisms and amphetamine abnormal behavior. Acta Pharmacol. Tox. 20: 145-157, 1963.

Ritvo, E.R., Yuwiller, A., Geller, E., Ornitz, E.M., Saeger, K. and Plotkin, S.: Increased blood serotonin and platelets in early infantile autism. Arch. Gen. Psychiat. 23: 566-572, 1970.

Robinson, D.S., Davis, J.M., Nies, A., Colburn, R.W., Davis, J.N., Bourne, H.R., Bunney, W.E., Shaw, D.M. and Coppen, A.J.: Ageing, monoamines and monoamine-oxidase levels. Lancet 1: 290-291, 1972.

Rosenberg, D.E., Isbell, H. and Miner, E.J.: Comparison of placebo, N-dimethyltryptamine, and 6-hydroxy-N-methyltryptamine in man. Psychopharmacologia 4: 39-42, 1963.

Rosenberg, D.E., Isbell, H., Miner, E.J. and Logan, C.R.: The effect of N,N-dimethyltryptamine in human subjects tolerant to lysergic acid diethylamide. Psychopharmacologia 5: 217-227, 1964.

Rosengarten, H., Szemis, A., Piotrowski, A., Romaszewka, K., Matsumato H., Stencka, K. and Jus, A.: N,N-dimethyltryptamine and bufotenin in the urine of patients with chronic and acute schizophrenic psychoses. Psychiatria Polska 4: 519-521, 1970.

Rothlin, E.: Pharmacology of lysergic acid diethylamide and some of its related compounds. In Psychotropic Drugs, ed. by S. Garattini and V. Ghetti, pp. 36-37, Elsevier Publishing Co., Amsterdam, 1957.

Saavedra, J.M. and Axelrod, J.: Psychotomimetic N-methylated tryptamines: formation in brain _in vivo_ and _in vitro_. Science 175: 1365-1366, 1972a.

Saavedra, J.M. and Axelrod, J.: A specific and sensitive enzymatic assay for tryptamine in tissues. J. Pharmacol. Exp. Ther. 182: 363-369, 1972b.

Saavedra, J.M., Coyle, J.T. and Axelrod, J.: The distribution and properties of the nonspecific N-methyltransferase in brain. J. Neurochem. 20: 743-752, 1973.

Sai-Halász, A.: The effect of antiserotonin on the experimental psychosis induced by dimethyltryptamine. Experientia 18: 137-138, 1962a.

Sai-Halász, A.: The role of serotonin antagonism in the model psychoses. (Hung.) Ideggyogy-Szemle 15: 301-305, 1962b.

Sai-Halász, A.: The effect of MAO inhibition on the experimental psychosis induced by dimethyltryptamine. Psychopharmacologia 4: 385-388, 1963.

Schatz, R., Ashcraft, E.A. and Sellinger, O.Z.: The elevation by methionine sulfoximine of rat brain histamine methyltransferase and catechol-O-methyltransferase activity. Trans. Am. Soc. Neurochem. 5: 184, 1974.

Schatz, R., Diez Altares, M.C. and Sellinger, O.Z.: Effect of methionine (MET) and methionine sulfoximine (MSO) on rat brain S-adenosyl methionine (SAM). Trans. Am. Soc. Neurochem. 4: 74, 1973.

Schwartz, M.A., Aikens, A.M., Neff, N.H. and Wayatt, R.J.: MAO activity in brains from schizophrenics and others. New Research Abstracts, p. 26, American Psychiatric

Association, Annual Meeting, Detroit, May, 1974a.

Schwartz, M.A., Aikens, A.M. and Wyatt, R.J.: Monoamine oxidase activity in brains from schizophrenic and mentally normal individuals. Psychopharmacologia 38: 319-328, 1974b.

Schwartz, M.A., Wyatt, R.J., Yang, H-Y.T. and Neff, N.H.: Multiple forms of brain monoamine oxidase in schizophrenic and normal individuals. Arch. Gen. Psychiat. 31: 557-560, 1974c.

Seevers, M.H. and Deneau, G.A.: Physiological aspects of tolerance and physical dependence. In Physiological Pharmacology, Vol. 1 - Part A, ed. by W.S. Root and F.G. Hofmann, pp. 565-640, Academic Press, New York, 1963.

Shapiro, S.K., Almenas, A. and Thomson, J.F.: Biosynthesis of methionine in Saccharomyces cerevisial. Kinetics and mechanism of reaction of S-adenosylmethionine: homocysteine methyltransferase. J. Biol. Chem. 240: 2512-2518, 1965.

Shulgin, A.T.: Personal communication, 1974.

Siegel, R.K. and Jarvik, M.E.: Hallucinogen induced responses in mice: Measurement and analysis. Abstract Fifth Int. Congress on Pharmacology, July 23-28, 1972.

Sloan, J.W., Martin, W.R., Clements, T.C., Bridges, S.R. and Buchwald, W.F.: Brain levels of tryptamine (T) in the cat, dog, guinea pig and rat. Fed. Proc. 33: 468, 1974.

Smythies, J.R. (ed.): The Mode of Action of Psychotomimetic Drugs. A Report Based on an NRP Work Session. Neurosciences Research Program Bulletin 8: 1, 152, 1970.

Smythies, J.R., Beaton, J.M., Benington, F. and Morin, R. D.: The design of some new compounds to block psychotomimetic drugs. Eur. J. Pharmacol. 17: 270-272, 1972.

Snyder, S.H.: CNS stimulants and hallucingens. In Chemical and Biological Aspects of Drug Dependence, ed. by S.J. Mulé and H. Brill, pp. 55-63, CRC Press, Cleveland, 1972.

Sourkes, T.L.: Alpha-methyltryptophan and its actions on tryptophan metabolism. Fed. Proc. 30: 897-903, 1971.

Sprintz, H., Parker, C.M., Jameson, D. and Alexander, F.: Urinary indoles in schizophrenic and psychoneurotic patients after administration of tranylcypromine (Parnate) and methionine or tryptophan. J. Nerv. Ment. Dis. 137: 246-251, 1963.

Swiatek, K.R., Simon, L.N. and Chao, K.L.: Nicotinamide methyltransferase and S-adenosylmethionine: 5l-methylthioadenosine hydrolase. Control of transfer ribonucleic acid methylation. Biochem. 12: 4670-4674, 1973.

Szára, S.: Dimethyltryptamin: Its metabolism in man; the relation of its psychotic effect to serotonin metabolism. Experientia 12: 441-442, 1956.

Szára, S.: The comparison of the psychotic effect of tryptamine derivatives with the effects of mescaline and LSD-25 in self-experiments. In Psychotropic Drugs, ed. by S. Garattini and V. Ghetti, pp. 460-467, Elsevier Publishing Co., Amsterdam, 1957.

Szára, S.: Hallucinogenic amines and schizophrenia. In Amines and Schizophrenia, ed. by H.E. Himwich, S.S. Kety and J.R. Smythies, pp. 181-197. Pergamon Press, Oxford, 1967.

Szára, S.: Hallucinogenic effects and metabolism of tryptamine derivatives in man. Fed. Proc. 20: 885-888, 1961.

Szára, S. and Axelrod, J.: Hydroxylation and N-demethylation of N,N-dimethyltryptamine. Experientia 15: 216-217, 1959.

Szára, S., Hearst, E. and Putney, F.: Metabolism and behavioral action of psychotropic tryptamine homologues. Int. J. Neuropharmacol. 1: 111-117, 1962.

Szasz, T.A.: Medicine and Madness. 1974 Britannica Book of the Year, pp. 454-455. Encyclopaedia Britannica, Inc., Chicago, 1974.

Tedeschi, D.H., Tedeschi, R.E. and Fellows, E.J.: The effects of tryptamine on the central nervous system, including a pharmacological procedure for the evaluation of iproniazid-like drugs. J. Pharmacol. Exp. Ther. 126: 223-232, 1959.

Tenen, S.S.: An automated one-way avoidance box for the rat. Psychonom. Sci. 6: 407-408, 1966.

Thithapandha, A.: Substrate specificity and heterogeneity of N-methyltransferase. Biochem. Biophys. Res. Comm. 47: 301-308, 1972.

Todrick, A., Tait, A.C. and Marshall, E.F.: Blood platelet 5-hydroxytryptamine levels in psychiatric patients. J. Ment. Sci. 106: 884-890, 1960.

Utena, H., Kanamura, H., Suda, A., Nakamura, R., Machiyama, Y. and Takahashi, R.: Studies on the regional distribution of monoamine oxidase activity in the brains of schizophrenic patients. Proc. Japan Acad. 44: 1078-1083, 1968.

Uzunov, P. and Weiss, B.: Psychopharmacological agents and the cyclic AMP: system of rat brain. In Advances in Cyclic Nucleotide Research, Vol. 1, pp. 435-453, Raven Press, New York, 1972.

Vasko, M., Lutz, M.P. and Domino, E.F.: Structure activity relations of some indolealkylamines in comparison to phenethylamines on motor activity and acquisition of avoidance behavior. Psychopharmacologia 36: 49-58, 1974.

Vogel, W.H., Orfei, V. and Century, B.: Activities of enzymes involved in the formation and destruction of biogenic amines in various areas of human brains. J. Pharmacol. Exp. Ther. 165: 196-203, 1969.

Walker, R.W., Ahn, H.W., Mandel, L.R. and VandenHeuvel, W.J.A.: Identification of N,N-dimethyltryptamine as the product of an in vitro enzymatic methylation. Anal. Biochem. 47: 228-234, 1972.

Walker, R.W., Ahn, H.S., Albers-Schonberg, G., Mandel, L.R. and VandenHeuvel, W.J.A.: Gas chromatographic-mass spectrometric isotope dilution assay for N,N-dimethyltryptamine in human plasma. Biochem. Med. 8: 105-113, 1973.

Weil-Malherbe, H. and Szára, S.I.: The Biochemistry of Funtional and Experimental Psychoses. C.C. Thomas, Springfield, 1971.

Weinshilboum, R.M. and Axelrod, J.: Reduced plasma dopamine-β-hydroxylase activity in familial dysautonomia. N. Engl. J. Med. 285: 938-942, 1971.

Wetterberg, L., Åberg, H., Ross, S.B. and Fröden, Ö.: Plasma dopamine-β-hydroxylase activity in hypertension and various neuropsychiatric disorders. Scan. J. Clin. Lab. Invest. 30: 283-289, 1972a.

Wetterberg, L., Gustavson, K.H., Bäckström, M., Ross, S.B. and Fröden, Ö.: Low dopamine-β-hydroxylase activity in Down's syndrome. Clin. Genet. 3: 152-153, 1972b.

Wise, C.D. and Stein, L.: Dopamine-β-hydroxylase deficits in the brains of schizophrenic patients. Science 181: 344-347, 1973.

Wise, C.D. and Stein, L.: Evidence of a central noradrenergic deficit in schizophrenia. In Neurotransmitter Balances Regulating Behavior, ed. by E.F. Domino and J. Davis, 99-123, Ann Arbor, Michigan, 1975.

Wooten, G.F., Eldridge, R., Axelrod, J. and Stern, R.S.: Elevated plasma dopamine-β-hydroxylase activity in torsion dystonia. N. Engl. J. Med. 288: 284-287, 1973.

Wyatt, R.J., Erdelyi, E., DoAmaral, J.R., Elliott, G.R., Renson, J. and Barchas, J.D.: Tryptoline formation by a preparation from brain with 5-methyltetrahydrofolic acid and tryptamine. Science 187: 853-855, 1975a.

Wyatt, R.J., Gillen, J.C., Kaplan, J., Stillman, R., Mandel, L.R., Ahn, H.S., VandenHeuvel, W.J.A and Walker, R.W.: DMT - A possible relationship to schizophrenia. Advances in Biochemical Psychopharmacology 11: 299-318, Serotonin-New Vistas, ed. by E. Costa, G.L. Gessa, and M. Sandler, Raven Press, New York, 1974.

Wyatt, R.J., Mandel, L.R., Ahn, H.S., Walker, R.W. and VandenHeuvel, W.J.A.: Gas chromatographic-mass spectrometric isotope dilution determination of N,N-dimethyltryptamine concentrations in normals and psychiatric patients. Psychopharmacologia 31: 265-270, 1973a.

Wyatt, R.J., Murphy, D.L., Belmaker, R., Cohen, S., Donnelly, D. and Pollin, W.: Reduced monoamine oxidase activity in platelets: A possible genetic marker for vulnerability to schizophrenia. Science 179: 916-918, 1973b.

Wyatt, R.J., Saavedra, J.M. and Axelrod, J.: A dimethyltryptamine forming enzyme in human blood. Amer. J. Psychiat. 130: 754-760, 1973c.

Wyatt, R.J., Schwartz, M.A., Erdelyi, E. and Barchas, J. D.: Normal dopamine-β-hydroxylase activity in the brains of chronic schizophrenic patients. Science 187: 368-369, 1975b.

Wyatt, R.J., Termini, G. and Davis, J.M.: Biochemical and sleep studies in schizophrenia: A review of the literature 1960-1970, Parts I and II. Schizophrenia Bull. 4: 10-66, 1971.

Wyatt, R.J., Vaughan, T., Galanter, M., Kaplan, J. and Green, R.: Behavioral changes of chronic schizophrenic patients given L-5-hydroxytryptophan. Science 177: 1124-1126, 1972.

Yang, H.-Y.T. and Neff, N.H.: The monoamine oxidases of brain: selective inhibition with drugs and the consequences of the metabolism of the biogenic amines. J. Pharmacol. Exp. Ther. 189: 733-740, 1974.

Zappia, V., Zydek-Cwick, C.R. and Schlenk, F.: The specificity of S-adenosylmethionine derivatives in methyl transfer reactions. J. Biol. Chem. 244: 4499-4509, 1969.

Neurotransmitter Balances Regulating Behavior,
edited and published by E.F. Domino and
J.M. Davis, Ann Arbor, © 1975

NEURONAL MODELS OF TRANSMITTER BALANCE

Steven Matthysse
Department of Psychiatry
Harvard Medical School
Boston, Massachusetts

Using neuronal models, I would like to suggest some of the ways in which transmitter balance might be brought about in the nervous system. These "lollipop neuron" models should not be taken too literally, in view of the complexity of the real nervous system, but they will serve their purpose if they alert us to the variety of possibilities for transmitter balance.

Our conceptual formulation of transmitter balance has gone beyond the classical ergotropic - trophotropic notions because we are no longer constrained to think of transmitters only as forces that can push in opposite directions. For example, stabilization of one transmitter system by another is a possibility illustrated in this circuit.

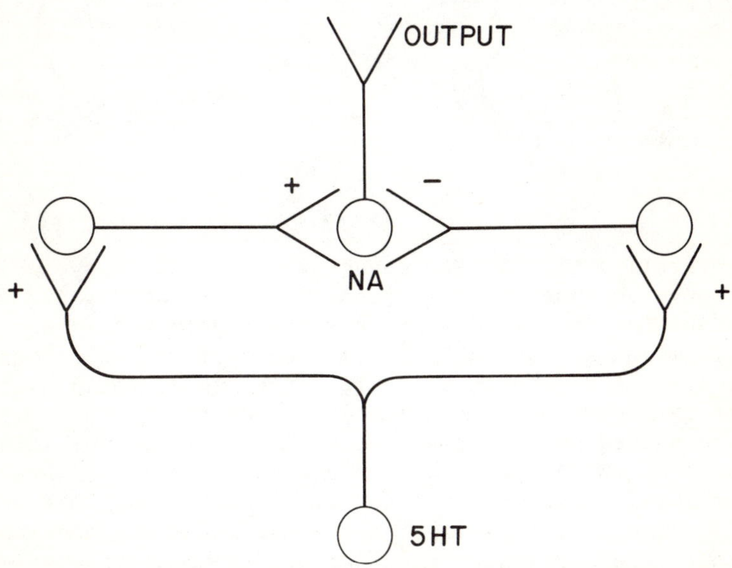

If we assume that the noradrenergic input is excitatory but insufficient by itself to fire the output neuron, its efficacy will depend on the fluctuations in membrane potential. If the other excitatory and inhibitory inputs to this neuron shown in the figure both fire at a high rate, the average membrane potential may not change, but the fluctuations will diminish (because of the statistical law of large numbers). Increased serotonin activity would, therefore, stabilize the effector pathway of this system against deviations in noradrenergic firing rate. Such a circuit could account for the relationships postulated by Kety between these transmitters in the modulation of affect; serotonin depletion permits mood swings but noradrenaline level controls their direction.

Alternatively, the relationship between serotonin and noradrenaline in the control of affect could be accounted for by a feedback circuit like this:

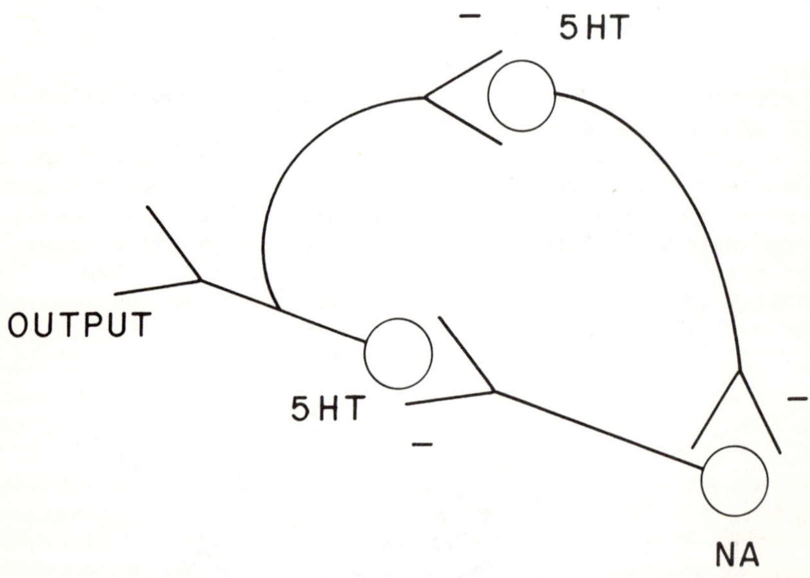

The overall action of the feedback control pathway is inhibitory, because $(-1)^3$ is negative. Serotonin would serve to stabilize the noradrenergic system against fluctuations but it might not directly influence the level of effector activity. A serotonin blocker, for example, would disinhibit the interneuron but its increased firing rate might not be passed on to the noradrenaline cell as inhibition because of the blockade of the second serotonin synapse. Conversely, an agent which facilitates serotonin actions would decrease the firing rate of the interneuron but potentiate the postsynaptic effect of its impulses on the noradrenergic neuron. These effects might cancel each other out. The stability of the feedback system against changes in activity of the noradrenaline cell would, however, be increased by agents which potentiate serotonin and be decreased by serotonin blockers.

The data presented on acetylcholine effects raises the interesting question of symmetry in the cholinergic system. According to Domino's experiments, acetylcholine agonists and antagonists act symmetrically with respect to self-stimulation behavior; physostigmine suppresses self-stimulation, anticholinergics facilitate it. On the other hand, with respect to mood, they seem to act asymmetrically: physostigmine acts as a depressant (Janowsky) but pure anticholinergics are not considered to be mood-elevating. This situation is similar to release of luteinizing hormone. According to McCann, atropine blocks LH release but carbachol does not release LH effectively. In contrast, the noradrenaline system seems generally to exhibit symmetry between agonists and antagonists. The lack of symmetry might be accounted for by postulating that there are cholinergic neurons involved in the control of mood which have low spontaneous activity. Facilitating agents would then have wide scope for their actions whereas inhibiting agents could only reduce the activity a small amount. The opposite assumption, high spontaneous activity with maximal receptor stimulation, would have to be assumed to prevail in the luteinizing hormone system.

Finally, I would like to suggest a model of dopaminergic-cholinergic interaction which may account for some of the more puzzling aspects of the pharmacology of schizophrenia. Davis and Janowsky have observed that physostigmine antagonizes methylphenidate-induced exacerbation of schizophrenia. On the other hand, physostigmine is not a therapeutic agent for naturally-occurring schizophrenia, and anticholinergics do not interfere with the therapeutic effects of phenothiazines. The absence of symmetry in these effects of cholinergic drugs is hard to reconcile with a simple "push-pull" balance theory. The following model, based on a mixture of the principles discussed above, does account for these observations. The overall effect of the feedback loop is inhibitory, as discussed before. Let us suppose that the pathological defect in schizophrenia is tonic hyperpolarization of the cholinergic interneuron so that it does not discharge. The cause could be a disturbed excitatory-inhibitory balance of other afferents to the interneuron not indicated in the diagram, or some defect in the interneuron itself. Using this model, we can account for the asymmetries in dopaminergic-cholinergic balance in the following way.

Physostigmine potentiates the action of acetylcholine, but in the schizophrenic there is nothing to potentiate, since the interneuron is silent. Methylphenidate inhibits the dopamine-receptive neuron, and therefore indirectly excites the cholinergic interneuron. After methylphenidate treatment, therefore, the situation has changed and the interneuron is firing, so physostigmine can potentiate its inhibitory control of the dopaminergic neuron. Phenothiazines excite the dopamine-receptive neuron by blocking inhibitory synaptic input, and therefore indirectly inhibit the cholinergic interneuron. The interneuron was not firing before the inhibition, so it is certainly not firing now; therefore, anticholinergics have nothing to block.

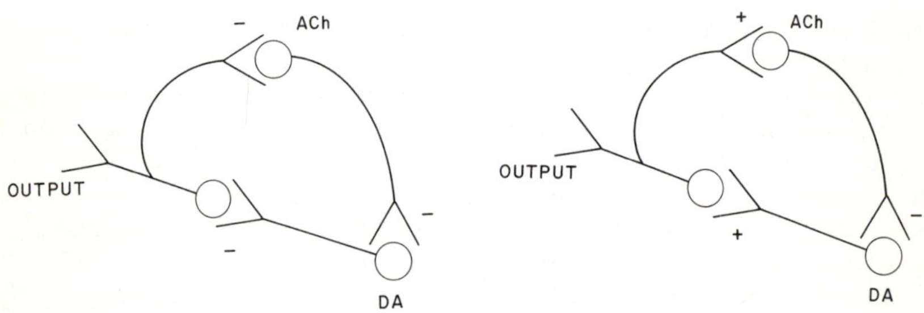

Peripheral receptors could be blocked with N-methylatropine, although central muscarinic receptors would be affected nonselectively. It has recently been reported that atropine, locally injected into the substantia nigra, increases neostriatal dopamine turnover, in contrast with its effects when administered systemically (Javoy et al., 1974). This observation is in accord with the model. It is possible to design a single circuit which is consistent with the local and systemic effects of atropine on dopamine turnover, the blocking effect of GABA antagonists on feedback inhibition, and the observations on "balance" discussed above. The feedback loop would have to be rather complex, containing two cholinergic neurons and one GABA neuron. The first cholinergic neuron would receive inhibitory dopaminergic input and would inhibit the second cholinergic neuron. The second cholinergic neuron would project downward, making excitatory connections with gabaminergic cells, which finally would inhibit the ascending dopamine neurons. The feedback properties of this system depend on several unknown parameters, but if the values are chosen appropriately, the observations referred to can be accounted for. Definitive modelling, of course, must await further neuroanatomical-neurochemical exploration of the descending pathway.

References

Javoy, F., Agid, Y., Bouvet, D. and Glowinsky, J.: Changes in neostriatal DA metabolism after carbachol or atropine microinjections into the substantia nigra. Brain Res. 68: 253-260, 1974.

INDEX